T0224982

Clinical Chinese Named Entity Recognition in Natural Language Processing

Shuli Guo · Lina Han · Wentao Yang

Clinical Chinese Named Entity Recognition in Natural Language Processing

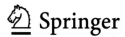 Springer

Shuli Guo
National Key Lab of Autonomous
Intelligent Unmanned Systems
School of Automation
Beijing Institute of Technology
Beijing, China

Wentao Yang
National Key Lab of Autonomous
Intelligent Unmanned Systems
School of Automation
Beijing Institute of Technology
Beijing, China

Lina Han
Department of Cardiology
The Second Medical Center
National Clinical Research Center
for Geriatric Diseases
Chinese PLA General Hospital
Beijing, China

ISBN 978-981-99-2664-0   ISBN 978-981-99-2665-7 (eBook)
https://doi.org/10.1007/978-981-99-2665-7

This Springer imprint is published by the registered company Springer Nature Singapore Pte Ltd.
The registered company address is: 152 Beach Road, #21-01/04 Gateway East, Singapore 189721,
Singapore

We heartily congratulate Prof. Si Ligeng of Inner Mongolia Normal University for his 90th birthday.

Preface

The topic about *Clinical Chinese Named Entity Recognition in Natural Language Processing* has a significant meaning for the progress in medicine. Our team has done some work about "Elderly health services and remote health monitoring" under the grant "National Key R&D Program of China" since August 2017. Professor Han and I have discussed every detail and tried our best to keep our desires coming true as soon as possible. The research work is divided into different parts according to the subject similarity and can help the readers to conduct in-depth and open research.

The aim of named entity recognition (NER) is to extract entities with actual meaning from massive unstructured texts. In the clinical and medical domains, clinical NER recognizes and classifies medical terms in unstructured medical text records, including symptoms, examinations, diseases, drugs, treatments, and operations. As a combination of structured and unstructured texts, the rapidly growing biomedical literature contains a significant amount of useful biomedical information. Moreover, NER is a key and fundamental part of many natural language processing (NLP) tasks, including the establishment of a knowledge graph, question and answer system, and machine translation. Therefore, Chinese NER (CNER) can extract meaningful medical knowledge to support medical research and treatment decision-making.

It is well known that software sciences are interesting but arduous subjects. This book aims to make software sciences lighter and easier to understand. Hopefully, this book is enjoyable for all readers. This book will help practitioners have more concise model systems for software techniques, which have the potential applications in the future world.

This book will be a valuable guide for researchers and graduate students in the fields of medicine management and software engineering.

Beijing, China

Shuli Guo
Lina Han
Wentao Yang

Acknowledgements

We wish to thank many professors who have given us comments concerning these topics in this book and those friends who have encouraged us to carry it out over the years. It is difficult to do anything in life without the friends' help, and many of my friends have contributed much to this book.

Our sincere gratitude goes especially to the Academician of the Chinese Academy of Sciences, Prof. Huang Lin of Peking University, Prof. Irene Moroz of Oxford University, President and Academician of the Chinese Academy of Engineering, Prof. Chen Jie of Tongji University, President and Academician of the Chinese Academy of Engineering, Fu Mengyin of Nanjing University of Science and Technology, Prof. Wang Long of Peking University, Prof. Cao Xiankun of Education Department of Hainan Province, Prof. Ren Fujun of China Association for Science and Technology, Prof. Fan Li, Prof. He Kunlun, Director Li Tianzhi, Director Li Xingjie, Prof. Wang Chunxi, Prof. Luo Leiming of Chinese PLA General Hospital, and Prof. Ma Wanbiao of University of Science and Technology, Beijing.

We wish to thank our colleagues and friends Prof. Wang Junzheng, Prof. Wu Qinghe, Prof. Xia Yuanqing, Prof. Wang Zhaohua, Prof. Zhang Baihai, Prof. Liu Xiangdong of Beijing Institute of Technology, Prof. Wei Yingbin of Hainan University, and Prof. He Jinxu of Hainan College of Software Technology.

We wish to thank our graduate Ph.D. degree students Song Xiaowei, Wang Guowei, Wang Hui, Wu Lei, Zhao Zhilei, Wu Yue, Cekderi Anil Baris and our graduate master degree students Zhao Yuanyuan, Guo Yanan, Li Qiuyue, Zhang Yating, and Yan Biyu.

We wish to thank Hainan Province Science and Technology Special Fund under the Grant ZDYF2021GXJS205 and Beijing Natural Science Foundations under the Grant M21018. We warmly celebrate Hainan College of Software Technology for his 100th birthday.

We also wish to take this opportunity to thank Dr. Huang Shuting of Dalian University of Technology for critically reviewing the entire manuscript and giving constructive comments on our manuscript.

We are truly indebted to Mr. Wayne Hu for working with me for 3 months to take care of the typing and preparation of this book's manuscript. Lastly, this book is dedicated to Mr. K. Rammohan and his colleagues for their active efforts.

Beijing, China   Shuli Guo
December 2022   Lina Han
                                                                                    Wentao Yang

Introduction

Entity recognition is an important task in NLP and has been made great progress in recent years. Natural language texts in the medical field, such as medical textbooks, medical encyclopedias, clinical cases, medical journals, hospital admission records, and test reports, contain a large amount of medical expertise and medical terminology. Applying entity recognition technology to medical expertise can significantly improve the efficiency and quality of clinical research. Automatic information processing from medical texts using machines can also serve downstream tasks such as medical knowledge mapping, diagnosis classification, drug-drug interaction (DDI), and adverse drug events (ADE) detection.

This book focuses on this topic in three areas:

- Enhancing the context capture capability of the model;
- Improving the location information perception capability of the pre-trained model;
- Denoising the recognition of unannotated entities in medical named entities.

Its specific contents have the following three areas.

(1) To improve the long short-term memory (LSTM) neural network model, this work improves the long-range dependency problem and the contextual information capture capability of the LSTM by adding a parameter-sharing unit to the LSTM. The proposed parameter-sharing unit cell contains both shared parameters that can be learned from the task and trained across a certain sequence length. Therefore, the proposed LSTM variant neural network with parameter sharing has a greater improvement in recognizing medical entities in long texts across a wider range of contexts and with richer text information.

(2) To strengthen the location information perception capability of bidirectional encoder representation from transformers (BERT) and to study the effect of the self-attention mechanism on location information, this work uses the method of Chinese sub-word grid results to modify the transformer, enhances the ability of model to learn location information, and then reduces its weakness for location information. Based on this goal, this work proposes a multilayer soft location matching format transformer entity auto-extraction model, aiming to select the best sub-word result by this work and soft location matching scores. Then this work uses the multi-grained

word grid to directly introduce a location representation for the transformer through the word and word sequence information. The transformer utilizes the fully connected self-attention to learn long-distance dependencies in sequences.

(3) To address the noise in the NER task due to the characteristics of the medical dataset itself, this work uses positive-unlabeled (PU) learning, a combination of negative sampling and pre-trained models, to reduce the impact of noise on the model. This work proposes a method that uses PU learning and negative sampling to train unlabeled entities and eliminate the errors caused by unlabeled entities, thus reducing the dependence of the model on text annotation.

Contents

About the Authors

Prof. Shuli Guo was born in 1973 in Inner Mongolia, P.R. China. He received his bachelor's degree (1995), master's degree (1998) from Inner Mongolia Normal University, and his Ph.D. degree from Peking University (2001). He worked as a postdoctoral researcher from January 2002 to April 2004 at Tsinghua University, as a researcher fellow from January 2008 to September 2008 at Akita Prefectural University, and as a postdoctoral researcher from September 2008 to September 2009 at Oxford University. His research interests include classical control theory and application, medical image processing, medical data analysis, typical chronic disease analysis, and remote medical monitoring. Recently, he has published nearly 70 impactful papers, three monographs, 34 authorized Chinese patents, 15 authorized software copyrights. He has published three Chinese national standards and handed in nine Chinese national standards/industrial standards for approval. He obtained one-third prize for military medical achievements, one-third prize of science and technology of the Chinese Medical Association, and one-third prize of Beijing Medical Science and Technology. And he is the member of Chinese national technical committee for professional standardization (2021–2026), the head of China geriatric disease standardized diagnosis and treatment society of CAGG (2018–2023), and the chief expert of Chinese national key research and development program (2017–2021).

Prof. Lina Han was born in 1973 in Jilin Province, P.R. China. She received her medicine bachelor's degree (1995), medicine master's degree (2000), and Ph.D. degree (2003) from Jilin University. She worked as a postdoctoral researcher from July 2003 to April 2005 at Chinese PLA General Hospital and as a research fellow from August 2008 to September 2009 at Kyoto University. And now, she works as a research fellow in Department of Cardiovascular Internal Medicine, National Clinical Research Center for Geriatric Diseases, The 2nd Medicine Center of Chinese PLA General Hospital, and Chinese PLA Medical School. Her research interests focus on many 3D modeling problems on cardiovascular systems and their medical solutions.

Mr. Wentao Yang was born in 1990 in Hebei Province, P.R. China. He received his bachelor's degree (2019) from Tianjin Institute of Technology and master's degree (2022) from Beijing Institute of Technology. His main research interests are the area of wireless sensor networks and software engineering.

Acronyms

ADE	Adverse Drug Event
Bert	Bidirectional Encoder Representation from Transformers
BiLSTM	Bidirectional Long Short-Term Memory Network
BioNER	Biomedical Named Entity Recognition
CBOW	Continuous Bag of Words
CNER	Chinese Named Entity Recognition
CNN	Convolutional Neural Network
CoVe	Contextualized Word Vectors
CRF	Conditional Random Field
DDI	Drug-Drug Interaction
EHR	Electronic Health Record
ELom	Embedding From Language Models
EM	Expectation Maximization Algorithm
FLAT	Flat-Lattice Transformer
FN	False Negative
FP	False Positive
Glove	Global Vectors for Word Representation
GRU	Gated Recurrent Unit
HMM	Hidden Markov Model
LSTM	Long Short-Term Memory
MLM	Masked Language Model
MNER	Medical Named Entity Recognition
MTL	Multi-Task Learning
NER	Named Entity Recognition
NLP	Natural Language Processing
NSP	Next Sentence Prediction

RNN	Recurrent Neural Network
SVM	Support Vector Machine
TN	True Negative
TP	True Positive
UMLS	Unified Medical Language System

Chapter 1
Theoretical Basis

1.1 Research Purposes

The aim of NER is to extract entities with actual meaning from massive unstructured text [1]. In the clinical and medical domain, clinical NER recognizes and classifies medical terms in unstructured medical text records, including symptoms, examinations, diseases, drugs, treatments, operations, and body parts. As a combination of structured and unstructured texts, the rapidly growing biomedical literature contains a significant amount of useful biomedical information. Moreover, NER is a key and fundamental part of many NLP tasks, including the establishment of a knowledge atlas, question answering system, and machine translation. Therefore, clinical NER can extract meaningful medical knowledge to support medical research and treatment decision-making.

Recently, there has been renewed interest in various medical and biomedical tasks, such as protein–protein interaction [2], DDI extraction [3], and chemical-protein interaction extraction [4, 5]. The objection of these tasks is to recognize entities and extract possible meaningful relations between them. For example, extracting pivotal knowledge about previously prescribed treatments or drugs and obtaining the relationship among treatments, drugs and diseases can be helpful to support decision-making [6]. Most of these tasks require two steps. First, medical entities mentioned in a given text are recognized by NER technologies. Next, the relation of each entity pair is categorized into the group required by tasks [7]. For medical information mining from unstructured text data in clinical records, NER is a crucial step, and the NER results may affect the performance of these tasks.

For the application of medical name recognition, initially, the approaches of establishing well-designed keyword search, rule-based systems [8], and feature sets [9] can usually achieve good performance. Nevertheless, the construction of the list of keywords and rules requires much manual work. Supervised machine learning [9] models have become a way to solve this problem and perform better than unsupervised approaches. However, their performance highly depends on the quality of annotated data.

© The Author(s), under exclusive license to Springer Nature Singapore Pte Ltd. 2023
S. Guo et al., *Clinical Chinese Named Entity Recognition in Natural Language Processing*, https://doi.org/10.1007/978-981-99-2665-7_1

As deep learning advances, deep learning for NER based on word embedding has gradually become popular [10]. LSTM with a conditional random field (CRF) [11, 12] is a typical deep learning modelling for NER that can learn similar representations for semantically or functionally similar words and can effectively extract features of text data. Although these deep learning models can significantly reduce resource consumption and manual labeling costs, they have a drawback that the embedding of the same word in varying semantic contexts is identical.

Recently, NLP has entered the era of pretrained models. Transformer [13], embedding from language models (ELom) [14], and BERT [15] in many NLP tasks have achieved current state-of-the-art results. The above models can learn structural information of language and generate more effective word representations from large-scale unannotated data in trained model than those only from limited annotated data. Then, these pretrained models are applied to CNER tasks by fine-tuned strategies.

For example, Biomedical Named Entity Recognition (BioBERT) [16] is a typical pretrained BERT. In pretraining, PubMed and PubMed Central (PMC) publications are used to train the vanilla BERT. Although BioBERT has a similar architecture with BERT, it contains rich linguistic information about the pretrained biomedical corpus. Thus, BioBERT achieved state-of-the-art results on the following three biomedical text tasks, including biomedical NER [17]. However, this work cannot encompass the entire language biomedical and clinical entity normalization tasks, especially Chinese which has no space between characters.

While the BERT model can generate a BERT embedding of English and overcome the limitations of traditional embedding that cannot capture the ambiguity, the pretraining of BERT corrupts the input and magnifies the sparsity of the data, and the BERT embedding obtained from training corpora with scarcity is likely to accomplish the tasks well. Some representative related approaches and previous studies are listed below. In the early stages of medical NER development, the common NER approach was mostly manually crafted expert rules, dictionaries, and heuristics to identify entities of interest. These rule-based approaches are still applied today, but they have drawbacks as follows. Many rules are required to maintain optimal performance, and text cannot automatically learn text based on text federation, which is vulnerable to data limitations and therefore lacks portability and robustness. Hence, the hidden Markov model (HMM) [18], maximum entropy Markov model (MEMM) [19] and CRF have become classic CNER methods that can solve sequence labeling problems. However, based on traditional machine learning, NER highly relies on feature selection, and suffers from a lack of generalizability. Moreover, their computation is expensive and has data sparsity issues [20].

In recent years, with the increase in computing power, NER based on deep neural networks has been able to solve these problems and is receiving more attention. In particular, the bidirectional LSTM with a CRF layer (BiLSTM-CRF) has less artificial conduction than rule-based methods and is powerful in capturing the potential relationship between the token and the cue. Wang et al. [21] proposed a BiLSTM-CRF BioNER combined multitask learning framework to solve NER. Yoon et al. [22] proposed CollaboNet to reduce false positives via multiple LSTM with CRF. Wunnava et al. [23] employed a BiLSTM-CRF to recognize and exact ADEs and had excellent extraction accuracy. Zhang et al. [24] proposed Lattice-LSTM by improving the internal structure of LSTM, which directly connected the embedding of the Chinese character and Chinese word to improve CNER based on correspondence.

These methods based on BiLSTM-CRF focus on feature extraction between words, but they do not have general-purpose priors and need to be trained from the beginning for specific tasks. With the Google BERT pretraining model proposed, this problem is overcome. Several CNER studies [25] used the outputs of the BERT model as word embedding and then input these BERT embeddings into the traditional BiLSTM-CRF model. The advantage of this approach is that it handles lexical ambiguity through combination with context.

Current researchers mainly focused on pretrained BERT on a large clinical unlabeled corpus, which achieved the optimal performance on extracting the named entities and relations of these entity pairs from the encounter notes, operation records, pathology notes, radiology notes, and discharged summaries of patience [26]. Li et al. [27] took a BERT-based model that was easily fine-tuned to normalize the types of entities and clinical terms and outperform them on the MADE 1.0 corpus compared with other models.

The studies mentioned above all use Recurrent Neural Network (RNN) and LSTM as the core to obtain contextual information to complete the NER task. However, LSTM, as a sequence model, cannot be computed in parallel, resulting in a long training time. Therefore, it is the focus to propose a method that can be computed in parallel and still has the function of LSTM to capture contextual information effectively. Therefore researchers started to focus on the use of Convolutional Neural Network (CNN) in CNER, such as Residue Dilated (RD)-CNN-CRF [28] and Dilated (ID)-CNN [29]. However, CNN needs to incorporate more convolutional layers in order to obtain contextual information, and leads to many hyperparameters of the network and still requires longer computation time.

However, most NER methods often take a long time for training and are unable to perform parallel computing. Motivated by the recent success of transformer and BERT approaches in dealing with various NLP tasks, the following methods are utilized in this work:

(1) A novel model is introduced based on pretrained BERT from the Chinese clinical corpus of NER, which enables to model information about Chinese characters and words. The experimental results show that this proposed method has high accuracy on the NER task.
(2) A novel selection scheme of word separation result is introduced, such as soft term position lattice, which can utilize lexical information to select lexical location information to locate the entity span.
(3) Novel soft lattice structure transformer layers are presented to build a simple and efficient module that can select more correct words and capture the contextual information during NER training.

1.2   Future Directions

1.2.1   Trends in Research and Development

As the core of hospital medical information systems, electronic medical records have always been important patient treatment data. The data integrity and path traceability of electronic medical records can effectively reduce medical errors and improve medical quality and safety. Therefore, NER is widely used in a large number of electronic medical records as an information processing method to automatically extract medical entity information from medical records. To some extent, NER can be regarded as a sequence tagging problem. Most of the current researches on NER have focused on building or improving models and evolving training methods on high quality annotated data. However, the models developed in these studies are weak in perceiving the information in the data. Therefore, this work aims to optimize the ability of model to acquire information from the data, and to improve the model adaptability to the NER task by inputting more informative word embeddings into the pretrained model through various embedding methods.

1.2.2   Long-Distance Dependencies

The issue of long-distance dependency was firstly discussed by Hockett in 1952, and Chomsky's Ph.D. thesis in 1957 discussed the input of long-distance dependency and their relationship with language theory through personal psychology. Based on the language, the meaning of a word is determined by the location of the word and the words surrounding it, and this is the information that NLP models learn word dependent information.

In the field of NLP, long-term dependency refers to the state of the current system, which may be influenced by the state of the system a long time ago, and is a problem that cannot be solved in RNNs. In medical nomenclature recognition, the most commonly used models based on RNN or LSTM are limited by gradient disappearance and the inability to span large segments of language. Some current researches have shown that the use of auxiliary information can alleviate the gradient problem and the problem of contextual information. Therefore, how to enhance the ability of LSTM to capture contextual information has become the focus of research.

1.2.3   Location Information Awareness Capability

When extracting entities from electronic health records (EHRs), NER models predominantly employ LSTM, and have shown impressive performance and results in clinical NER. The reason for such good results in NER is that LSTM models can often increase the depth of the network to capture long-range dependencies. Because of this, these time-series neural network-based LSTMs typically require long training times and large amounts of training data to achieve high accuracy, which hinders the adoption of LSTM-based models in clinical scenarios where training time is limited. Therefore, building a model that both captures contextual information and enables parallel computation with less computation time becomes the future research goal.

BiLSTM has been widely used as encoders for NER tasks. Recently, fully connected self-attentive architectures (aka Transformer) have been widely used for various NLP tasks due to their parallelism and advantages in remote context modelling. However, the performance of the vanilla Transformer in NER is not as good as other NLP tasks. The reasons are as follows: on one hand, the Transformer adopts a self-attentive mechanism and does not model the context sequentially as LSTM does, instead computes word attention at different locations, and therefore does not learn positional information.

1.2.4   Dataset Noise Problem

It is difficult to label many of the data with negative samples because real-life samples of well-labeled data may not always be available. Then the negative data samples are so diverse and dynamic that they can lead to a large number of unlabeled positive samples in the training data.

For NLP, the lack of data is an important constraint that limits the training of models, especially in the field of biology and medicine, where medical naming entities involve numerous specialized terms and terminologies that require professional practitioners to annotate, which is time-consuming and costly, so the lack of data is currently a major problem faced by biomedical NER. Therefore, the use of remote supervision to solve the problem of insufficient data and data annotation has become a key direction in the field of NER research. However, remote supervision often leads to mislabelled data with a large amount of noise affecting the final performance of the model, for example, only 20% of samples belonging to a certain class are labelled in the dataset, while the remaining 80% mislabelled samples contain samples belonging to the former and not belonging to the later.

1.3   Purpose and Significance of the NER

As the core of the hospital medical information system, electronic medical records have always been important patient treatment data. The data integrity and path traceability of electronic medical records can effectively reduce medical errors and improve the quality and safety of medical treatment.

Therefore, NER, as an information processing method to automatically extract medical entity information from medical records, has been widely used in a large number of electronic medical records. NER can be regarded as a sequence tagging problem to a certain extent. Most of the current researches on NER have focused on building or improving models and evolving training methods on high quality annotated data, but less research has been conducted to improve NER performance by extracting more information from limited data sets. However, the models developed in the above studies are weak in perceiving the information in the data. Therefore, this work improves the model ability to acquire information from the data, and optimizes the model adaptability to the NER task by inputting word embedding containing more information into the pretrained model through various embedding methods.

NER belongs to the field of NLP and is a fundamental and critical task in NLP. With the proliferation of electronic medical records and health records data nowadays, NER is gradually playing an important role in many NLP tasks such as relationship extraction, event extraction, knowledge atlas, attribute extraction, question and answer systems, sentiment analysis, machine translation, etc., with a wide range of applications.

Therefore, for the rapid medical development, a huge amount of clinical medical knowledge exists as unstructured data in texts such as electronic medical records and health records, and at the same time the texts contain a large amount of rich relational knowledge about ADE and the diseases evolution, so NER has become one of the important ways to intelligently obtain information from the large amount of medical texts. In the past few years, great progress has been made in applying NER methods to clinical informatics research using NER. For example, medical NER is applied to the classification of medical terms extracted from EHR, where NER is used for computational phenotyping, diagnostic classification, novel phenotype discovery, clinical trial screening, pharmacogenomics, drug therapy, DDI, adverse effects, and the identification of medical conditions. DDI, ADE detection, and genome-wide and phenomenon-wide association learning. NER also plays a large role in the calculation of phenotypes. A phenotype is a characteristic expression of genotypic variation and interaction between an organism and its environment, consisting of physical appearance (e.g. height, weight, body mass index), biochemical processes or behaviors, and is usually summarized by experts based on clinical records and patient observations. The EHRs require for phenotype calculation which contains a large amount of digital health data and unstructured clinical narratives (e.g. progress notes and discharge summaries), unstructured clinical records or their combination to mine or predict clinically and scientifically phenotypes. Therefore, it is essential to use NER technology to analyse automatic structures of EHR data where phenotypes can be calculated. In addition, NER is also applied in medical intelligence management, such as medical information extraction, medical intelligent triage, clinical medical decision support, medical information management, medical automatic consultation, medical knowledge mining, medical knowledge atlas construction and so on.

For engineering applications of medical nomenclature recognition, an initially good performance can usually be achieved using well-designed keywords searches and rule-based systems. However, the construction of keywords and rule lists required significant manual efforts, so the use of supervised machine learning models is the solution to this problem, allowing classification patterns and structures to be obtained from the data. With the development of deep learning, the adoption of deep learning models for the NER task became the mainstream approach, deep neural networks is used to effectively extract features from text data, and resource consumption and manual annotation costs are greatly reduced. As NLP enters the pretrained era, pretrained models (e.g. ELmo, Transformer, Bert, etc.) for completing NER increasingly become widespread and show a promise in improving the NER performance. Often, better performances can be achieved by combining multiple information forms.

NER plays an important role in the NLP. NER aims to automatically discover words with important information in medical texts and to identify entities based on the context of the text. NER is simultaneously required to find the boundaries of entities and to accurately classify them. Typically, clinical NLP systems are developed and evaluated on word level, sentence level or document level. Model specific attributes and features are annotated, such as document contents (e.g. patient status or report type), types of document section (e.g. current medication, past medical history or discharge summary), named entities and concepts (e.g. diagnosis, symptoms or treatment) or semantic attributes (e.g. negation, severity or transience). Therefore, the attributes and features of medical texts effectively determine the performance of complex analytical systems such as medical knowledge atlases and decision support systems.

Rau's firstly published a paper titled "Extraction and Recognition of Company Names" at the 7th IEEE Conference on Applications of Artificial Intelligence in 1991, which is considered as the first presentation of NER. Since 1996, the NER has greatly become a sub-task of information extraction in academic conferences. For example, the named entity evaluation as an assigned-task of information extraction appeared MUC-6 international conference in 1996.

So far, the typical methods of biological NER have gone through stages of heuristic rule-based methods [30], lexical matching methods [31], machine learning methods and deep learning methods such as Support Vector Machine (SVM) [32], maximum entropy [33], HMM [34] and CRF [35], etc.

It is well known that the NER task initially required elaborate heuristic rules to identify the hits and a good accuracy has been achieved by modelling comprehensive rules to identify entity methods. For example, Tsuruoka [36] minimized the ambiguity and variability of terms in dictionaries by using a discovery style rule approach, that is to say that the standardization of names was used as a means in improving the efficiency of finding dictionaries. However, the heuristic rule approach is heavily dependent on some domain knowledge and even the integrity of the designed the rules. Especially, designing the rules and modifying the rules require the involvement of experts in the scene and considerable time to design the rules and more importantly strengthen in migration and generalization. Simultaneously, the rule-based approach difficultly copies with the emergence of new entities and the diversity of named entity types, but also difficultly continues to emerge a consistent set of rules. Currently, rule-based methods are applied to NER tasks, and acted as decoders in the NER post-processing by using machine learning methods.

Other methods that have emerged alongside rule-based methods are been applied to NER tasks include dictionary-based methods, which are first used by Proux [37] and others in 1998 to identify gene and protein entities using English dictionaries. This method uses dictionary matching to achieve entity identification, but it is poor in following aspects such as identifying new entities or variants of entities as the dictionary which does not contain new named entities, building comprehensive and extensive entity coverage and completing dictionaries of named entities in medical biology. As a result, dictionary-based methods are gradually being fused by machine learning methods with better performance. Some current researches still focus on entity recognition in the form of dictionary features, but mainly in the form of combination with machine learning methods [38].

Currently, some methods based on machine learning are commonly used, moreover machine learning uses statistical methods to estimate relevant parameters of engineering feature from large amounts of data and thus build recognition models. Machine learning in NER is mainly divided into classification models, sequence annotation models and so on. On one hand, NER modeling can be seen as a word classification problem by firstly vectorizing features or texts and then using classification-based methods such as Bayesian models and SVMs; on the other hand, NER modeling can also be seen as a sequence labelling problem due to the sequence information of textual terms (both utterances and sequences of labeled utterances), so CRFs, Markov-based models, HMMs, and so on can be used.

Statistical-based machine learning methods use statistical algorithms and artificial set features to train the model, which are divided into the following steps such as feature selecting, classification designing and post-processing. Machine learning models are more flexible and can be slow because of the large amount of data and the complexity of model.

1.4 Current Status and Trends

1.4.1 Research Trends

Early medical NER methods mainly use rule-based methods, which require experts in specialized fields to manually design rules based on their accumulated medical knowledge, and often consume a lot of manpower and time costs, with high costs and poor portability, in this way rule-based methods are not being widely used. Subsequently, machine learning methods rely more on engineering features, so their generalization ability remains limited. With the development of deep learning methods and their applications on NER, the advantages of deep learning models such as efficiently automatically extracting features through designed networks are gradually apparent. Deep learning differs from machine learning, which avoids the tedious process of extracting features and reduces manual involvement. Due to such advantages of deep learning, the applications of deep learning models in BioNER have become an interesting hot. The mainstream neural networks for NER adopt LSTM, among which the joint of LSTM and CRF gets outstanding results on NER. For example, the Highway-LSTM-CRF model was constructed by Zhao [39]. With the widespread use of attention mechanism in neural networks, the BiLSTM-Attention-CRF [40] model has become the mainstream NER method.

For BioNER dealing with multidimensional English, NER mostly uses word embedding techniques based on English representations, while for medical selection of specific word embedding methods, such as Wikipedia, Common Crawl or specific pretrained embedding methods in biomedical literature, it provides better embedding results through modeling. Simultaneously, the Unified Medical Language System (UMLS) [41] will be tried to the medical naming recognition. This is because the NER approaches fusing with UMLS have numerous following advantages. Firstly, the meta-synonymy database of UMLS contains the core data table of UMLS, which has concepts and terms derived from different source word lists and also integrates the conceptual relationships existing in different source word lists; in terms of data quality, it not only facilitates the completion of NER tasks, but also does the implementation of other natural language tasks based on NER, such as relationship extraction, knowledge atlas, etc. Moreover, the semantic network of UMLS [42] forms semantic relations between concepts by assigning semantic types to all integrated concepts, and these semantic relations form a semantic network of concepts, each of which may have one or more semantic types, and can play the role of medical disambiguation and semantic annotation, and much do disambiguation and data enhancement; finally, for the terminological variants faced by a named body recognition and the problem of terminological variants faced in nomenclature recognition, the problem of terminological variants can be effectively solved by using the expert dictionary of UMLS, which contains various variants of terms related to pathology, anatomical entities, biochemical or pharmacological substances, diagnostic or therapeutic procedures, laboratory tests as well as processes, and avoid high variability of medical entities and terms. In addition, the UMLS support software package is very convenient and facilitates the development and use of UMLS.

In terms of Chinese medical nomenclature entity recognition, it is characterized by a dense distribution of Chinese entities in the text, especially in medical texts (e.g. electronic medical records), which is twice as dense as that of ordinary Chinese texts, and it simultaneously faces the problem of accuracy due to the dense entity distribution, but it is also the dense entity distribution that makes Chinese text data more valuable for research. To address the problem of dense entity distribution affecting recognition accuracy, Chinese researchers have utilized the following three approaches to medical nomenclature recognition, namely inputting more features to deep learning models, incorporating other machine learning, and making improvements to the model structure. For example, multi-feature embedding, word embedding fusion embedding, location information [43] or using the characteristics of Chinese pictographs to encode radicals as features [44, 45] are used to improve the recognition of NER. In addition to fusing more features, methods such as migration learning [46], joint learning and Multi Task Learning (MTL)

[47], and reinforcement learning [48] are also beginning to be applied to NER tasks. In terms of the NER model structure improvement, Flat-Lattice-Transformer (FLAT) [49] by Xipeng Qiu's team at Fudan University in 2020 is an approach that uses the NER model structure to improve the long-term dependencies of multiple sequences via Transformer Encoder. Although NER has been developed for many decades and numerous advances have been made, it is still facing challenges such as complex extraction, small sample customized extraction, noise-reduced extraction, cross-language extraction, multimodal extraction, and open extraction. In response, to address the problem of noise reduction extraction brought about by the lack of training data or mislabelling, the Tencent AI team use the following two methods for noise reduction, namely changing the annotation framework and negative sampling of non-entities [50].

1.4.2 Previous Research Work

In medical nomenclature recognition, the most commonly used deep models fall into two main categories. One class is RNN or LSTM models, but RNN-based approaches suffer from two limitations such as the gradient disappearance and the inability to span large segments in the problem of language spanning. Another class of approaches is based on Transformer or BERT models, but suffers from a weak ability to capture contextual location information.

For LSTM or RNN based on NER, Pesaranghader's BioWSD [51] model is based on a BiLSTM deep learning model that uses text definitions from the UMLS for word disambiguation purposes, while suffers from the long distance dependency limitation of BiLSTM. Norgeot [52] has created the largest corpus of manually annotated clinical notes for the protected health information and the developed Philter, a customizable open source de-identification software. Wang [21] used a MLT framework to obtain multiple models by the BioNER model with firstly training data containing different types of entities and then sharing the training model parameters, thus alleviating the NER limitation problem brought by the small number of available entity types. Yoon [22] proposed CollaboNet based on MLT and multiple NER models in order to reduce the impact of insufficient data and the multiplicity of biological entities on the effectiveness of entity type classification.

Wunnava [23] developed a rule-based sentence and a word tokenization technique for adversing drug event detection, through providing well-labelled textual input as a way to reduce noise in EHR text, and doing a three-layer deep learning architecture of recurrent neural networks for ADE detection methods. The character-level word representation utilizes BiLSTM through the integration of different word embedding methods, i.e. the above two sequence tagging techniques to fuse each other and a two-layer embedding to represent character-level and word-level in the input layer. Wei [53] used a BiLSTM-CRF model approach to extract drugs and associated ADEs from clinical documents. The above studies are still implemented with BiLSTM-CRF as the main model and face the long-distance dependence deficit due to the limitations of LSTM itself.

Giorgi [54] used deep learning and migration learning to enhance the limited data to improve NER recognition through transfer knowledge and data augmentation. During the process of recognition, embedding vectors are defined as tandem word embeddings and character embeddings, and two different bidirectional RNNs sharing output with the LSTM accomplish two different tasks such as lexical tagging and NER. The above two tasks are trained alternatively so that the knowledge from the lexical tagging task can be used to improve the performance of the NER task. Bhatia [55] proposed a hierarchical encoder-decoder NER model to coextract entities and discover negative and positive discrimination, firstly using a shared encoder based on the RNN and then separating decoders for the coextraction and discrimination. Wang [56] well accomplished domain transfer for NER models with multiple types of data by using shared and private domain parameters and a MLT approach. However, the model is still unable to improve the long-range dependency deficit of BiLSTM. The above researches and developments all use knowledge-based data augmentation methods, aiming to improve the performance of deep learning models for biomedical NLP by overcoming the scarcity of training data to achieve good recognition results. Among them, the UMLS-based recognition of English medical named entities has also emerged as a knowledge augmentation approach. For example, UMLS-EDA effectively improves deep learning models for NER and sentence classification and can provide novel information for resource-poor biomedical domains, offering unique insights into deep learning methods.

In terms of utilizing Transformer or BERT for NER tasks, Zhang [57] used unlabeled EHR to fine-tune BERT as a way of constructing an MC-BERT model, which performed well in standardizing medical and clinical entities. In order to address the feature of low generalization, the biomedical domain requires comprehensive multi-platform medical data for training data, then transferring different data to complete the NER task, however, there is a risk of privacy exposure. Simultaneously, Transformers or BERT on the NER task also have the disadvantage of weak location awareness, and Yan [58] improved Transformer for the NER task with a simple amelioration of the attention scoring function to enhance Transformer's ability to capture location information.

With BERT [59] making a splash in the field of NLP, some NER research has also turned its attention to Bert. Lee [16] pretrained BERT on a large biomedical corpus to obtain the biomedical domain language representation model BioBERT, which solves the transferring model from a general domain corpus to a biomedical one for text mining. By pretraining on the large biomedical corpus and fine-tuning it to suit the NLP task, BioBERT far outperforms pretrained BERT in the general domain on many biomedical text mining tasks, and demonstrates great advantages on the NER task. Zhang [26] used a fine-tuned pretrained bi-directional encoder in the BERT model to extract concepts and their attributions from clinical breast cancer documents. The approach consists of two components: a NER component and a relationship recognition. For the NER component, BERT is fine-tuned to achieve NER, and the method outperforms other methods on the NER task. Peng [60] proposed a MLT model with multiple decoders for a variety of biomedical and clinical NLP tasks, such as text similarity, relation extraction, NER and text inference. MTL, together with BERT, is used for multiple biomedicine and NER.

From the above studies based on the pretrained model BERT, it can be seen that BERT enables further performance improvements on biomedical entity recognition and clinical entity normalization, because BERT can be easily fine-tuned to normalize and recognize any kind of named entities, and to migrate strongly. However, the above Transformer or BERT-based models still suffer from the weak ability to capture contextual location information.

Therefore, Chinese NER (CNER) research has started to make use of lexical augmentation, with the idea of combining information from dictionaries to improve CNER. CNER based on lexical augmentation mainly adopts a dynamic framework to be compatible with lexical input and to construct adaptive word vectors. On one hand, among the lexical enhancement methods using dynamic frameworks, Lattice LSTM fused all word information of the current character through the word unit structure [61], but Lattice LSTM causes information loss, poor transferability and long training time; LR-CNN [62] and LGN [63] used global information to introduce lexical information losslessly, and CGN [64] constructs a collaborative graph network-based model to introduce lexical information for lexical enhancement. On the other hand, among the adaptive word embedding approaches, Word Character-LSTM (WC-LSTM) [65] and Multi-digraph [66] used different strategies to model characters and lexicon, but they also suffered from information loss. In response, Soft-lexicon [67] used BMES tags to fuse the representation information of the current character and their lexical collections, which caused no information loss while being portable, but relied on word embeddings.

For the denoising remote supervision problem, PU learning is an important method for denoising data samples. Since well-labelled data samples may not always be available in real life, many data labelling negative class samples is more difficult. Secondly, the negative class data samples are too diverse and dynamically changing, which tends to result in a large number of unlabelled positive samples in the training data. PU learning was first used in recommender systems, in which user clicks to be considered as positive samples, but because the position of the clicked sample may be inaccurate, the model cannot identify whether the unclicked user is a negative or positive sample, resulting in unmarked positive samples.

PU learning methods are divided into integrated learning style and two-step learning, where Spy-Expectation Maximation (S-EM) algorithm identifies non-negative samples by mixing positive and negative sample techniques to form a data set and then uses the classifier to train through data that is accurately labelled as negative samples. Cosine-Rocchio [68] used the similarity of positive samples from unlabelled samples and the named Cosine-Rocchio classification method to construct the classifier, resulting in a final reliable negative example. The Positive Example Based Learning (PEBL) algorithm [69] used a 1DNF approach to form word sets from positive words that occurred more frequently in the unlabelled set, and then negative word sets from subsets of the unlabelled set did not contain any positive words in the word set. In addition, PU learning also makes use of different classification models, for example, the EM-Naive Bayesian EM-NB [70] uses a positive sample set and a negative sample set to construct a Parsimonious Bayesian classifier, and then applies the Parsimonious Bayesian classifier to classify each sample in the negative sample set, finally obtains the set of samples predicted to be negative samples. The SVM-iteratively with classifier selection (IS) [71] bases on three types set such as the set of positive samples, the set of samples classified as negative, and the set of missing categories (i.e., the intersection of the set of negative samples and the set of samples predicted as negative). In each iteration, a new SVM classifier is correspondingly constructed from the set of positive samples and the set of samples classified as negative samples, and then the new SVM classifier is applied to classify the documents in the missing category set. The set of documents classified as negative is removed from the missing category set and added to the set of samples classified as negative. The iteration stops when no documents in the missing category set are classified as negative. However, so far, PU learning has seldom been applied to the NER task. The reason is that the entity recognition is difficult in achieving reliable sample sets, but building and using reliable entity dictionaries lead to error propagation and affect the final classification results.

In summary, current medical NER methods are either recurrent neural network and LSTM network models, or Transformer and BERT models, but LSTM suffers from the problem of weak ability to capture contextual location information. Meanwhile, Transformer or BERT studies cannot fully improve gradient disappearance and inability to span large segments of language. Therefore, the noise of data from Chinese medical entities is difficult to solve.

The organizational framework of this book is shown in Fig. 1.1.

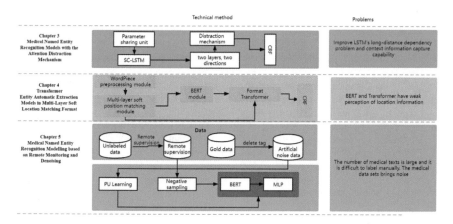

Fig. 1.1 Organizational framework of this book

References

1. Zhang Q, Sun Y, Zhang LL, Jiao Y, Tian Y. Named entity recognition method in health preserving field based on BERT. Procedia Comput Sci. 2021;183:212–20.
2. Zhang YJ, Lin HF, Yang ZH, Wang J, Sun YY. Chemical-protein interaction extraction via contextualized word representations and multihead attention. Database. 2019. https://doi.org/10.1093/database/baz054.
3. Asada M, Miwa M, Sasaki Y. Using drug descriptions and molecular structures for drug–drug interaction extraction from literature. Bioinformatics. 2021;37:1739–46.
4. Luo L, Yang Z, Cao M, Wang Y, Zhang HL. A neural network-based joint learning approach for biomedical entity and relation extraction from biomedical literature. J Biomed Inform. 2020;103: 103384.
5. Hong L, Lin J, Li S, Wan F, Yang H, Jiang T, Zhao D, Zeng J. A novel machine learning framework for automated biomedical relation extraction from large-scale literature repositories. Nat Mach Intell. 2020;2:347–55.
6. Casillas A, Ezeiza N, Goenaga I, Pérez A, Sotor X. Measuring the effect of different types of unsupervised word representations on medical named entity recognition. J Biomed Inform. 2019;129:100–6.
7. Christopoulou F, Tran TT, Sahu SK, Miwa M, Ananiadou S. Adverse drug events and medication relation extraction in electronic health records with ensemble deep learning methods. J Am Med Inform Assoc. 2020;27:39–46.
8. Zhang SD, Elhadad N. Unsupervised biomedical named entity recognition: experiments with clinical and biological texts. J Biomed Inform. 2013;46:1088–98.
9. Settles B. Biomedical named entity recognition using conditional random fields and rich feature sets. In: Proceedings of the international joint workshop on natural language processing in biomedicine and its applications. Association for Computational Linguistics (NLPBA/BioNLP); 2004. p. 107–10.
10. Petasis G, Vichot F, Wolinski F, Paliouras G, Karkaletsis V, Spyropoulos C. Using machine learning to maintain rule-based named-entity recognition and classification systems. In: Proceedings of the 39th annual meeting of the Association for Computational Linguistics. 2001. p. 426–33.
11. Gong LJ, Zhang ZH, Chen SQ. Clinical named entity recognition from Chinese electronic medical records based on deep learning pretraining. J Healthc Eng. 2020. https://doi.org/10.1155/2020/8829219.
12. Ling Y, Hasan SA, Farri O, Chen Z, Ommering R, Yee C, Dimitrova N. A domain knowledge-enhanced LSTM-CRF model for disease named entity recognition. In: AMIA summits on translational science proceedings, vol. 761. 2019. 761–70.
13. Vaswani A, Shazeer N, Parmar N, Uszkoreit J, Jones L, Gomez AN, Kaiser Ł. Attention is all you need. Adv Neural Inf Process Syst. 2017;5998–6008.
14. Peters ME, Neumann M, Iyyer M, Gardner M, Clark C, Lee K, Zettlemoyer L. Deep contextualized word representations. 2018. arXiv preprint arXiv:1802.05365.
15. Devlin J, Chang MW, Lee K, Toutanova K. Bert: pre-training of deep bidirectional transformers for language understanding. 2018. arXiv preprint arXiv:1810.04805.
16. Lee J, Yoon W, Kim S, Kim D, Kim S, Ho CS, Kang J. BioBERT: a pre-trained biomedical language representation model for biomedical text mining. Bioinformatics. 2020;36(4):1234–40.
17. Khattak FK, Jeblee S, Pou-Prom C, Abdalla M, Meaney C, Rudzicz F. A survey of word embeddings for clinical text. J Biomed Inform. 2019;100:100057.
18. Morwal S, Jahan N, Chopra D. Named entity recognition using hidden Markov model (HMM). Int J Nat Lang Comput. 2012;1(4):15–23.
19. McCallum A, Freitag D, Pereira F. Maximum entropy Markov models for information extraction and segmentation. In: Proceedings of the seventeenth international conference on machine learning, vol. 17. 2000. p. 591–8.

20. Qin QL, Zhao S, Liu CM. A BERT-BiGRU-CRF model for entity re electronic medical records. Complexity. 2021;2021:1–11.
21. Wang X, Zhang Y, Ren X, Zhang Y, Zitnik M. Cross-type biomedical named entity recognition with deep multi-task learning. Bioinformatics. 2019;35(10):1745–52.
22. Yoon W, So CH, Lee J, Cai P. CollaboNet: collaboration of deep neural networks for biomedical named entity recognition. BMC Bioinf. 2019;20(10):55–65.
23. Wunnava S, Qin X, Kakar T, Sen C, Rundensteiner EA, Kong XN. Adverse drug event detection from electronic health records using hierarchical recurrent neural networks with dual-level embedding. Drug Saf. 2019;42(1):113–22.
24. Zhang Y, Yang J. Chinese NER using lattice LSTM. 2018. arXiv preprint arXiv:1805.02023.
25. Li XY, Zhang H, Zhou XH. Chinese clinical named entity recognition with variant neural structures based on BERT methods. J Biomed Inform. 2020;107: 103422.
26. Zhang X, Zhang Y, Zhang Q, Ren Y, Qiu TL, Ma JH. Extracting comprehensive clinical information for breast cancer using deep learning methods. Int J Med Informatics. 2019;132: 103985.
27. Li F, Jin YH, Liu WS, Rawat BPS, Cai PS, Yu H. Fine-tuning bidirectional encoder representations from transformers (BERT)-based models on large-scale electronic health record notes: an empirical study. JMIR Med Inform. 2019;7:14830.
28. Qiu J, Zhou YM, Wang Q, Ruan T, Gao J. Chinese clinical named entity recognition using residual dilated convolutional neural network with conditional random field. IEEE Trans Nanobiosci. 2019;18:306–15.
29. Yu F, Koltun V. Multi-scale context aggregation by dilated convolutions. 2015. arXiv preprint arXiv:1511.07122.
30. Fukuda K, Tamura A, Tsunoda T, Takagi T. Toward information extraction: identifying protein names from biological papers. Pac Symp Biocomput. 1998;707(18):707–18.
31. Tuason O, Chen L, Liu H, Blake J A, Friedman C. Biological nomenclatures: a source of lexical knowledge and ambiguity. Pac Symp Biocomput. 2004;238–49.
32. Bakir G, Hofmann T, Schölkopf B, Joachims T, Altun Y. Support vector machine learning for interdependent and structured output spaces. In: International conference on machine learning IMLS, Banff, Alberta. 2004. p. 104.
33. Lin YF, Tsai TH, Chou WC, Wu KP, Sung TY. A maximum entropy approach to biomedical named entity recognition. In: International conference on data mining in bioinformatics ICDMB. Tokyo: Springer; 2004. p. 56–61.
34. Su J, Su J. Named entity recognition using an HMM-based chunk tagger. In: Meeting on Association for Computational Linguistics. Taipei: Association for Computational Linguistics ACL; 2002. p. 473–80.
35. Lafferty J, McCallum A, Pereira FCN. Conditional random fields: probabilistic models for segmenting and labeling sequence data. In: The eighteenth international conference on machine learning ICML, Williamstown. 2001. p. 282–9.
36. Tsuruoka Y, Tsujii J. Boosting precision and recall of dictionary-based protein name recognition. In: Proceedings of the ACL 2003 workshop on natural language processing in biomedicine, vol. 13. 2003. p. 41–8.
37. Proux D, Rechenmann F, Julliard L, et al. Detecting gene symbols and names in biological texts a first step toward pertinent information extraction. Genome Inform. 1998;9:72–80.
38. Zeng Z, Deng Y, Li X, Naumann T, Luo Y. Natural language processing for EHR-based computational phenotyping. IEEE/ACM Trans Comput Biol Bioinf. 2018;16(1):139–53.
39. Zhao DY, Huang JM, Jia Y. Chinese name entity recognition using Highway-LSTM-CRF. In: Proceedings of the 2018 international conference on algorithms, computing and artificial intelligence ACAI, Sanya. 2018. p. 1–5.
40. Luo L, Yang Z, Yang P, Zhang Y, Wang L, Lin H. An attention-based BiLSTM-CRF approach to document-level chemical named entity recognition. Bioinformatics. 2018;34(8):1381–8.
41. Bodenreider O. The unified medical language system (UMLS): integrating biomedical terminology. Nucleic Acids Res. 2004. 32(suppl_1):D267–70.

42. Kang T, Perotte A, Tang Y, Ta C, Weng CH. UMLS-based data augmentation for natural language processing of clinical research literature. J Am Med Inform Assoc. 2021;28(4):812–23.
43. Yang T, Jiang D, Shi S, Zhan S, Zhuo L, Yin Y, Liang Z. Chinese data extraction and named entity recognition. In: 2020 5th IEEE international conference on big data analytics (ICBDA). IEEE; 2020. p. 105–9.
44. Bollegala D, Hayashi K, Kawarabayashi KI. Think globally, embed locally: locally linear meta-embedding of words. In: Proceedings of the 27th international joint conference on artificial intelligence. 2018. p. 3970–6.
45. Coates JN, Bollegala D. Frustratingly easy meta-embedding–computing meta-embeddings by averaging source word embeddings. In: Proceedings of NAACL-HLT. 2018. p. 194–8.
46. Lee JY, Dernoncourt F, Szolovits P. Transfer learning for named-entity recognition with neural networks. In: Proceedings of the eleventh international conference on language resources and evaluation (LREC 2018). 2018.
47. Guo S, Yang W, Han L, Song X, Wang G. A multi-layer soft lattice based model for Chinese clinical named entity recognition. BMC Med Inform Decis Mak. 2022;22:1–12.
48. Yang Y, Chen W, Li Z, et al. Distantly supervised NER with partial annotation learning and reinforcement learning. In: Proceedings of the 27th international conference on computational linguistics. 2018. p. 2159–69.
49. Li X, Yan H, Qiu X, Huang X. FLAT: Chinese NER using flat-lattice transformer. In: Proceedings of the 58th annual meeting of the Association for Computational Linguistics, online: ACL. 2020. p. 6836–42.
50. Li Y, Liu L, Shi S. Empirical analysis of unlabeled entity problem in named entity recognition. Int Conf Learn Representations. 2020;5(4):343–9.
51. Pesaranghader A, Matwin S, Sokolova M, Pesaranghader A. Deep BioWSD: effective deep neural word sense disambiguation of biomedical text data. J Am Med Inform Assoc. 2019;26(5):438–46.
52. Norgeot B, Muenzen K, Peterson TA, Fan XC, Glicksberg BS, Schenk G, Rutenberg E, Oskotsky B, Sirota M, Yazdany J, Schmajuk G, Ludwig D, Theodore GT. Protected health information filter (Philter): accurately and securely de-identifying free-text clinical notes. Nat Digit Med. 2020;3(1):1–8.
53. Wei Q, Ji Z, Li Z, Du J, Wang J, Xu J, Xiang Y, Tiryaki F, Wu S, Zhang Y, Tao C, Xu H. A study of deep learning approaches for medication and adverse drug event extraction from clinical text. J Am Med Inform Assoc. 2020;27(1):13–21.
54. Giorgi JM, Bader GD. Transfer learning for biomedical named entity recognition with neural networks. Bioinformatics. 2018;34(23):4087–94.
55. Bhatia P, Celikkaya B, Khalilia M. Joint entity extraction and assertion detection for clinical text. In: Proceedings of the 57th annual meeting of the Association for Computational Linguistics ACL, Florence. 2019. p. 954–9.
56. Wang J, Kulkarni M, Preoţiuc-Pietro D. Multi-domain named entity recognition with genre-aware and agnostic inference. In: Proceedings of the 58th annual meeting of the Association for Computational Linguistics, online: ACL. 2020. p. 8476–88.
57. Zhang N, Jia Q, Yin K, Dong L, Gao F, Hua N. Conceptualized representation learning for Chinese biomedical text mining. 2020. arXiv preprint arXiv:2008.10813.
58. Yan H, Deng B, Li X, Qiu X. TENER: adapting transformer encoder for named entity recognition. Comput Sci. 2019;342–441.
59. Kenton JDMWC, Toutanova LK. BERT: pre-training of deep bidirectional transformers for language understanding. In: Proceedings of NAACL-HLT. 2019. p. 4171–86.
60. Peng Y, Chen Q, Lu Z. An empirical study of multi-task learning on BERT for biomedical text mining. In: Proceedings of the 19th SIGBioMed workshop on biomedical language processing, online: ACL-BioNLP-WS. 2020. p. 205–14.
61. Zhang Y, Yang J. Chinese NER using lattice LSTM. In: Proceedings of the 56th annual meeting of the Association for Computational Linguistics EMNLP-IJCNLP, Hong Kong, vol. 1. 2018. p. 1554–64.

62. Gui T, Ma R, Zhang Q, Zhao L, Jiang Y, Huang X. CNN-based Chinese NER with lexicon rethinking. In: The 28th international joint conference on artificial intelligence IJCAI, Macao. 2019. p. 4982–8.
63. Gui T, Zou Y, Zhang Q, Peng M, Fu J, Wei Z, Huang X. A lexicon-based graph neural network for Chinese NER. In: Proceedings of the 2019 conference on empirical methods in natural language processing and the 9th international joint conference on natural language processing EMNLP-IJCNLP, Hong Kong. 2019. p. 1040–50.
64. Sui D, Chen Y, Liu K, Zhao J, Liu S. Leverage lexical knowledge for Chinese named entity recognition via collaborative graph network. In: Proceedings of the 2019 conference on empirical methods in natural language processing and the 9th international joint conference on natural language processing EMNLP-IJCNLP, Hong Kong. 2019. p. 3830–40.
65. Liu W, Xu T, Xu Q, Song J, Zu Y. An encoding strategy based word-character LSTM for Chinese NER. In: Proceedings of the 2019 conference of the North American chapter of the Association for Computational Linguistics: human language technologies NAACL, Minneapolis, vol. 1. 2019. p. 2379–89.
66. Ding R, Xie P, Zhang X, Lu W, Li L, Si L. A neural multi-digraph model for Chinese NER with gazetteers. In: Proceedings of the 57th annual meeting of the Association for Computational Linguistics ACL, Florence. 2019. p. 1462–7.
67. Ma R, Peng M, Zhang Q, Huang X. Simplify the usage of lexicon in Chinese NER. In: Proceedings of the 58th annual meeting of the Association for Computational Linguistics, online: ACL. 2020. p. 5951–60.
68. Liu B, Lee W S, Yu P S, Li X. Partially supervised classification of text documents. In: The nineteenth international conference on machine learning ICML, Sydney, vol. 2(485). 2002. p. 387–94.
69. Li X L, Liu B, Ng SK. Negative training data can be harmful to text classification. In: Proceedings of the 2010 conference on empirical methods in natural language processing EMNLP, Stroudsburg. 2010. p. 218–228.
70. Yu H, Han J, Chang KCC. PEBL: web page classification without negative examples. IEEE Trans Knowl Data Eng. 2004;16(1):70–81.
71. Liu B, Dai Y, Li X, Xu Y, Peng T. Building text classifiers using positive and unlabeled examples. In: The third IEEE international conference on data mining. Melbourne: IEEE; 2003. p. 179–86.

Chapter 2
Related Existed Models

There are some related existed models of NLP such as Word Embedding, CRF, Deep Neural Networks et al. The simple and necessary introductions are listed as following.

2.1 Word Embedding

Word embeddings, also known as word representations, aim at transforming text words into digital vectors for representation, which include static embeddings such as One-Hot encoding, Word2Vec [1] (CBOW and SkipGram Models), Global Vectors for Word Representation (Glove) [2], and dynamic embeddings such as Contextualized Word Vectors (CoVe), ELom, Generative Pre-trained Transformer (GPT), BERT, Robustly Optimized BERT (RoBERT), Masked Sequence to Sequence Pre-Training (MASS), XLNet, Extensible Markup Language (XLM), Unified Language Model (UniLM).

2.1.1 One-Hot Encoding

One-Hot encoding is a sparse word representation originally used in the field of NLP, and is used for the digitization of nonnumerical features in the field of machine learning. For example, assuming that there are V distinct words, doxastic encoding represents a word as a vector with the length V. There is the 1st, ..., $V - 1$th zeros in the doxastic vector, and the Vth character or word has a doxastic encoding as 1 on the position. However, words, which are represented by the doxastic encoding way, do not represent the semantic similarity among words, and have large sparsity.

S. Guo et al., *Clinical Chinese Named Entity Recognition in Natural Language Processing*, https://doi.org/10.1007/978-981-99-2665-7_2

2.1.2 Word2Vec

The current popular word vector model is Word2Vec [1], which mainly converts words and phrases into high-quality distributed vectors containing semantic word relationships, also known as word embeddings, and its common approach consists of two main models such as the continuous bag of words (CBOW) model and the SkipGram model (SG). CBOW predicts the mask words based on the context window around it, and while SG is used to predict the possible adjacent words in the context window of a single input word. SG is applicable to scenarios with a few data, by more training samples can be constructed from a smaller data set. CBOW may construct one training sample of the central word based on the surrounding words, whereas SG constructs multiple training samples of the surrounding words based on the central word. Both are two-layer fully connected neural networks with linear activation in the hidden layer and a number of activation options in the output layer, whose activations from a softmax function produce a multinomial posterior distribution. For SG prediction, the output is the probability of predicting the target word, which results in each prediction being computed on the entire dataset, and requiring long training times, and producing less accurate embeddings. So those all require more space, Word2Vec is demanded to set layered softmax and negative sampling to speed up the training.

2.1.3 Glove

Glove is a global approach to word vectors obtained by matrix decomposition [2], that is to say, the co-occurrence matrix of words is first counted, whose element represents the number of times that word i and context word j occur together within a particular size context window. The rows or columns of the co-occurrence matrix are then used as word vectors. An approximate relationship between the word vector and the co-occurrence matrix is constructed through the following Eq. 2.1.

$$w_i^T \tilde{w}_j + b_i + \tilde{b}_j = \log(x_{ij}) \tag{2.1}$$

And at same time, the loss function is calculated based on the following relation 2.2.

$$J = \sum_{i,j=1}^{V} f\left(X_{i,j}\right)\left(w_i^T \tilde{w}_j + b_i + \tilde{b}_j - \log X_{i,j}\right) \tag{2.2}$$

where $Cove(\omega) = MT\text{-}LSTM(GloVe(\omega))$, which can be designed independently, is continuous at 0, not decreasing, and has an upper limit.

Glove can not only avoid the problem that the weight of high-frequency words is too large based on matrix decomposition, but also avoid the problem that the sliding window cannot get the data co-occurrence information. Glove applies the sliding context window to the training corpus and the construction of the co-occurrence matrix of the corpus range. The word embedding representation not only contains the statistical information of the global vocabulary, but also takes into account the local window context method. Compared with the global matrix decomposition method, the vocabulary with zero co-occurrence times is filtered out, the smaller of two matrices from the decomposition output is retained as the embedding matrix, and the above procedure reduces the computational load and data storage space. However, Glove is more sensitive to the number of corpora. When the number of corpora is relatively small, Glove cannot count the number of co-occurrences, which leads to the misleading of the word vector training direction.

2.1.4 CoVe

Within a lot of NLP work, there are a lot of polysemy, where the meaning of the same word needs to be judged according to the context, and so recognizing the meaning of words in context has become a research direction of word embedding. CoVe [3] is the original dynamic word embedding, which borrows from the idea of the deep network level to extract features of machine vision, and uses the deep LSTM to vectorize the text.

The context-dependent vector CoVe is used as the context vector through the output of LSTM-based machine translation model, with the relation Eq. 2.3.

$$\text{Cove}(\omega) = \text{MT-LSTM}(\text{GloVe}(\omega)) \qquad (2.3)$$

2.1.5 ELMo

ELMo [4] is trained on a language model with LSTM as the basic component to predict the next word in context. Through being trained from left to right, ELMo also is known as the autoregressive language model. ELMo creates a contextual representation of each tag by processing the static word vector by a two-layer LSTM, and then splices the internal state of each layer LSTM. That is to say, the first layer, the second layer and the third layer of the hidden vector are stitched together to get the complete context word vector containing the context of the word.

2.2   Conditional Random Fields (CRF)

CRF [5] is a common base model for processing label sequence criteria in NLP, and its function is to increase the rationality of label sequences. The CRF layer can make the final prediction label legal, and ensure the validity of the prediction results by adding some constraints. How to increase the constraints can be automatically learned by the CRF layer during the training process, which significantly reduces the generation of invalid predictive tag sequences. CRF, as a discriminant model, does not calculate the probability distribution, while calculates the final output. It has the characteristics of black box model, uses the feature functions to score different criteria, and then selects the most likely result according to the obtained scores.

For example, in the classic used BiLSTM-CRF model, the score of each tag can be obtained by the output of the BILSTM layer. The score of each tag will be used as the input of the CRF layer. CRF, which acts as a decoder, chooses the tag sequence with the highest score as the best solution.

For the given transformation score matrix A_{y_i-1,y_i} and the matrix p_{i,y_i} from the BiLSTM containing the probabilities of the labels y_j representing the words i, the CRF can calculate the scores of the sequences, where x denotes the sequence of sentences, y is the output sequence of labels, so the corresponding scoring function is defined as Eq. 2.4.

$$score(x, y) = \sum_{i-1}^{n} p_{i,y_i} + \sum_{i-1}^{n+1} A_{y_i-1y_i} \tag{2.4}$$

To make the transition matrix more stable, the START and END tags will be added, and finally the normalized probability can be obtained through the Softmax function.

$$p(y|x) = \frac{\exp(score(x, y))}{\sum_y \exp(score(x, y))} \tag{2.5}$$

The objective function or the optimization object of CRF can be calculated by Eq. 2.6, and the Viterbi algorithm is used to find the optimal path with the highest score.

$$y^* = \text{argmax}(score(x, y')) \tag{2.6}$$

2.3 Deep Neural Networks

2.3.1 Long Short-Term Memory (LSTM)

The LSTM is a variant of an RNN network that introduces gating mechanisms to alleviate the long dependence and gradient problems of RNN [6]. The LSTM has the same chain structure as RNN, but the difference from RNN is the operation logic inside each neuron with an optional memory unit.

The update model for its each unit and hidden output is Eq. 2.7.

$$
\begin{aligned}
f_t &= \delta\left(W_{fh}h_{t-1} + W_{fi}x_t\right) \\
i_t &= \delta(W_{ih}h_{t-1} + W_{ix}x_t) \\
o_t &= \delta(W_{oh}h_{t-1} + W_{ix}x_t) \\
c_t' &= \tanh(W_{ch}h_{t-1} + W_{cx}x_t) \\
c_t &= f_t * c_{t-1} + x_t * c_t' \\
h_t &= o_t * c_t
\end{aligned}
\tag{2.7}
$$

where x_t is an input, h_{t-1} is a hidden layer, f_t is a forgetting gate, c_t' is the memory unit of the current state of the input unit, and $*$ represents the Hadamard product with the multiplication of bits.

The memory of the LSTM at a given moment consists of two parts, the state information input at that moment and the state information input at the previous moment, which are not mandatory to be remembered. Both are values between 0 and 1 that can control the influence of the previous moment and the current moment on the current moment, and simultaneously both are automatically obtained by the network during training. The network solves the LSTM gradient problem by automatically adjusting the value of the corresponding gate to decide whether the gradient disappears or keeps. According to back-propagation, the gradient structure of the LSTM is spread to obtain the partial derivatives as in Eq. 2.8.

$$
\frac{\partial C_t}{\partial C_{t-1}} = \frac{\partial C_t}{\partial f_t}\frac{\partial f}{\partial h_{t-1}}\frac{\partial h_{t-1}}{\partial C_{t-1}} + \frac{\partial C_t}{\partial i_t}\frac{\partial i_t}{\partial h_{t-1}}\frac{\partial h_{t-1}}{\partial C_{t-1}} + \frac{\partial C_t}{\partial \tilde{C}_t}\frac{\partial \tilde{C}_t}{\partial h_{t-1}}\frac{\partial h_{t-1}}{\partial C_{t-1}} + \frac{\partial C_t}{\partial C_{t-1}}
\tag{2.8}
$$

$$
\frac{\partial C_t}{\partial C_{t-1}} = C_{t-1}\delta'(\cdot)W_f * o_{t-1}\tanh'(C_{t-1}) + \tilde{C}_t\delta'(\cdot)W_i * o_{t-1}\tanh'(C_{t-1})
$$
$$
+ i_t\tanh'(\cdot)W_c * o_{t-1}\tanh'(C_{t-1})
\tag{2.9}
$$

where the gate function gives the network ability to determine the extent to which the gradient vanishes, as well as the ability to set different values at each time step, and their values are set by the learning functions with respect to the current inputs and hidden states. In Eq. 2.9, the partial derivative is changed from a multiplicative to an additive operation, which avoids multiplication leading to the gradient vanishing after multiplication by zero, and updates additive unit states to make the derivative stable.

2.3.2 Transformers

The Transformer [7] framework adopts an encoder-decoder modeling framework with a Self-Attention mechanism at its core, which eschews the RNN-style sequential structure through updating contextual progress of hidden layer states and enhances the Transformer's parallelism. Meanwhile, using self-attentiveness and residual networks enhances the training speed, shortens the information distance and arbitrarily preserves long-term memory.

For Transformer, its multi-headed attention layer is composed of multiple parallel self-attentive mechanisms, which achieves an analogous CNN multi-channel mechanism that allows the model to extract data features in parallel.

While the encoder-decoder structure of the Transformer, the encoder inputs the sequence and processes it to obtain an intermediate representation, and then the decoder reads the obtained representation and processes it to form the varying length sequence output. Here the decoder consists of six sub-layers, which contains a multi-headed attention layer and a multi-layer perception layer with connecting mutually through the residual connection and the normalization layer. For facilitating the residual connectivity, the six sub-layer dimensions are all 512. The decoder layer are also designed to contain six sub-layers, which also has the same structure as the encoder layer, but with an additional multi-headed attention layer than the encoder layer. Their self-attention mechanisms are defined as Eqs. 2.10 and 2.11.

$$Attention(Q, K, V) = soft \max\left(\frac{QK^T}{\sqrt{d_k}}\right)V \tag{2.10}$$

$$[Q, K, V] = E_x\left[W_q, W_k, W_v\right] \tag{2.11}$$

where V represents the input features vector, Q, K are the feature vectors for calculating the attention weights, and E_x are all linear transformations from the input word vectors

$$i_t = \tanh\left[W_{cd}(r_t * d_{t-1})\right] = \tanh\left\{W_{cd}\left[r_t * (\delta(W_{rx}x_t + W_{rh}h_{t-1})\right]\right\},$$

where x_t are three linear variations to Q, K, V, and are obtained from the input features. Attention (Q, K, V) is the multiplication of V by the corresponding weights according to the degree of attention, and the similarity between the current word Q and all other words K is calculated according to Eq. 2.11 in the self-attentive mechanism, for the current word Q and all other words K. Through the Softmax layer, the maximum weight of the similarity between these current words and all other words is obtained. According to the product of the obtained maximum weight and the corresponding V value, the V value in the self-attention mechanism is obtained. So h_{t-1} makes the inner product not too large. Otherwise, when d_k is too large, the inner product correspondingly becomes large, which makes the gap between the inner product becomes too large, which results in the softmax's gradient very small. The above result is difficult in training the model for effective learning. While QK^T can guarantee the attention matrix as a normal distribution, it is advantageous to accelerate the convergence of the model.

Then, through the connection of the multi-headed attention mechanisms, a higher dimensional vector is firstly mapped into multiple lower dimensional vectors, thus the features of multiple perspectives are obtained, and then each perspective feature goes to realize the calculation of attention, so that the learning ability and potential of the whole model will be greatly enhanced, and in addition, because the dimensional reduction of the model is all parametric, it allows the whole model to learn the most useful perspectives based on the presented data.

The multi-headed attention model is shown in Eq. 2.12.

$$MultiHead(Q, K, V) = Concat(head_1, \ldots, head_n)W^O$$
$$head_i = Attention(QW_i^Q, KW_i^K, VW_i^V) \tag{2.12}$$

Since the self-attention does not have access to position information and always ignores the key information of sequence order, position embedding needs to be used to introduce position information. Specifically, some functions with different sin and cos periods are defined to calculate the embedding obtained for each position, as in Eq. 2.13.

$$PE(pos, 2i) = \sin\left(\frac{pos}{10,000^{\frac{2i}{d_{model}}}}\right)$$
$$PE(pos, 2i + 1) = \cos\left(\frac{pos}{10,000^{\frac{2i}{d_{model}}}}\right) \tag{2.13}$$

where d_t denotes the position of the word in the current sentence and W_{rx} is the index of each vector value. If the positions index W_{rx} is even, the sine function is adapted to encode, otherwise the cosine function is chosen to encode. The position encoding has the same 512 dimensions as the word embedding. And the word embedding and the above obtained position embedding are added to get the final word embedding.

For the residual connection network, the residual network connects the input and output results of the upper layer, and performs normalization, so as to alleviate gradient disappearance to a certain extent.

2.3.3   The Pretrained BERT Model

The BERT [8] model was proposed by Google in 2018, which consisted of the bi-directional structure Encoder in Transformer. And simultaneously its self-attention mechanism can parallelly realize the probability calculation of the current word, in the other words, the BERT model not only can make use of the contextual information, but also can speed up the calculation by using the parallelism of the self-attention mechanism.

The main highlight of BERT is to simultaneously use the two pretraining methods such as the masked language model (MLM) and the next sentence prediction (NSP), which use the following masking strategy to learn the semantic expressions of words. The masking strategy is as follows: when the BERT is trained, MLM pretraining strategy is used. For example, 15% of the words in the corpus are randomly masked, and the masking operation for these 15% words can also be divided into three cases.

(1)   MASK: 80% of the 15% words are directly replaced with the Mask;
(2)   REPLACE: 10% of 15% words are directly replaced with a new word;
(3)   KEEP: 10% of the 15% words remain unchanged.

When BERT comes to sentence-level tasks, such as question and answer systems and reading comprehension, it needs to learn sentence-level features and information. And at this time, the pretraining task is chosen to achieve these tasks through using the NSP, whose prediction goal is to learn the connection between two sentences. This is achieved by the pretraining inputs of sentences *A* and *B*, with a 50% chance that *B* is the next sentence of *A*. The inputs of these two sentences are used to predict whether *B* is the next sentence of *A* or not through the BERT model. In addition, the above models use *GELU* [9] activating the BERT model rather than the standard *RELU*, where the training loss is the sum of the average masked LM likelihood and the average NSP likelihood.

Since the time complexity of self-attention is the square of the length of the input sequence, a longer sequence will reduce the training speed, therefore, for the method of speeding up the pretraining in the experiment, the 90% sequence length is usually set to be 128, and the length of the remaining steps is set to 512.

2.4   The Task Description

2.4.1   The Purpose of the Task

NER itself is a combination of sequence annotation and phrase classification. Sequence annotation requires the classification of each word (Chinese character) or phrase contained in the sequence, because Chinese characters are the basic text unit in Chinese medical texts, but the entity is usually a phrase, which is a sequence of multiple characters, therefore, sequence annotation is the need to parse the tagging to get the boundary of the entity, and further get the category of the words.

The medical NER is essentially some medical sequence tagging, and the sequence tagging algorithm generally depends on the pre-and/or post-of the current word to consider the finite span of the sequence tagging. Learning a limited span of missing medical information reduces learning time, which also is the algorithm itself learning in a limited range of medical sequences, but NER is also easy to ignore valuable medical contextual information. Instead, this kind of sequence annotation classifies each entity (word or phrase) in the text sequence, and mainly extracts the boundary and category of the entity, as shown in Fig. 2.1.

At present, the standard format of the medical NER is mainly divided into two following types of BIO annotation and BIOES annotation.

- BIO annotation mode: B (Begin) represents the left boundary of the entity, I (Inside) does still the interior of the entity and O (Outside) does the outside boundary of the entity.
- BIOES annotation mode: "BIO" has the same meaning as the above BIO annotation mode, but the addition of E (End) represents the right boundary of the entity and S (Single) does the entity represented by a single character.

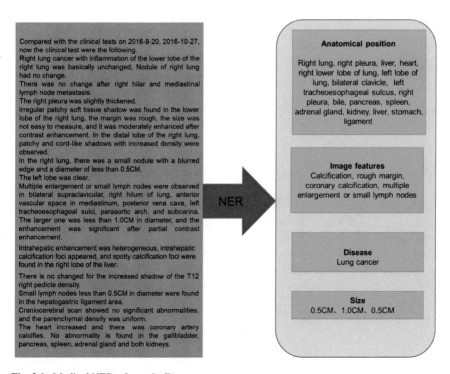

Fig. 2.1 Medical NER schematic diagram

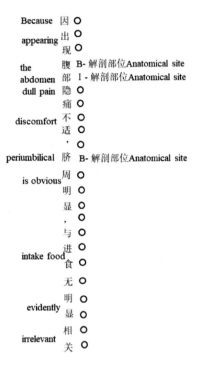

Fig. 2.2 BIOES annotation mode schematic diagram

In Chinese context, it is mainly marked by characters or phrases, but because Chinese does not have the same space as English and segmentation is difficult, the recognition accuracy cannot be guaranteed, so the current mainstream of CNER is BIO annotation in words. The identified entity types are diseases, image examination, tests, treatments, medicine, anatomy, and so on, as shown in Fig. 2.2.

2.4.2   The Problems of Chinese Named Entity Recognition

Firstly, Chinese does not have upper case letters and lower case letters, so CNER cannot get the entity information based on upper or lower case letters as English can, which is most obvious on NER.

Secondly, there are no spaces in Chinese. If a word-based sequence NER algorithm is adapted, which deals with the word segmentation, Chinese word segmentation will affect the final NER results. And Chinese word segmentation is still a difficult problem in Chinese NLP which cannot achieve a completely accurate effect, and there are always with certain errors.

2.4.3 The Characteristics of Chinese Medical NER

The Chinese clinical text is a clinical descriptive text written by the hospital doctor according to the image as well as test results, which contains complex information such as patient's basic conditions, medical history, medications, lifestyle habits, image descriptions, physical signs, indicators and so on. The fact written by different doctors leads to a certain degree of misspellings and errors in the clinical texts. Besides the presence of a large number of long terms, abbreviations and other words of more than five words in medicine, the mixing of Chinese and English also makes it difficult to identify medical named entities.

2.5 Evaluation Indexes

The evaluation indexes adopted in this book include the following, such as accuracy rate, precision rate, recall rate, F1 and confusion matrix. And the F1 evaluation index is still dominant, so as to reduce the influence of data imbalance on evaluation. As the NER task is a multi-classification task, the vertical columns and horizontal rows in the confusion matrix indicate the predicted classification results and the true classification results.

In the dichotomous task, True Positive (TP) indicates that the prediction is correct and the prediction is Positive, and the True category is also Positive; that is, correct classification being into positive. True Negative (TN) indicates that the prediction is correct and the prediction is Negative, the True category is also Negative; that is, correct classification being into negative.

False Positive (FP) indicates a prediction error, a Positive prediction, and the true category of the sample is negative, i.e. the negative case is incorrectly classified as a positive case.

False Negative (FN) indicates a prediction error, a Negative prediction, and the true category of the sample is positive, i.e. the positive case is incorrectly classified as a negative case. Based on the above four statistical concepts, Eqs. 2.14–2.17 define accuracy, precision, recall and F1, respectively.

$$Accuracy = \frac{TP + FN}{TP + FP + TN + FN} \tag{2.14}$$

$$Precision(P) = \frac{TP}{TP + FP} \tag{2.15}$$

$$Recall(R) = \frac{TP}{TP + FN} \tag{2.16}$$

$$F1 = 2 \cdot \frac{precision \cdot recall}{precision + recall} \tag{2.17}$$

For the evaluation of multi-categorical tasks, evaluation indicators for each category can be used and averaged, e.g. Macro-F_1.

It needs to be pointed out that the work's experiments are in Ubuntu 18.04 system, Python 3.8 programming language with depth framework for python, hardware environment for i7-9700k CPU, 32G memory, video card for RTX2080.

References

1. Mikolov T, Chen K, Corrado G, Dean D. Efficient estimation of word representations in vector space. 2013. arXiv preprint arXiv:1301.3781.
2. Pennington J, Socher R, Manning CD. Glove: global vectors for word representation. In: Proceedings of the 2014 conference on empirical methods in natural language processing EMNLP, Doha. 2014. p. 1532–43.
3. McCann B, Bradbury J, Xiong C, Socher R. Learned in translation: contextualized word vectors. Adv Neural Inf Process Syst. 2017;30:125–34.
4. Sarzynska-Wawer J, Wawer A, Pawlak A, Szymanowska J, Stefaniak I, Jarkiewicz M, Okruszek L. Detecting formal thought disorder by deep contextualized word representations. Psychiatry Res. 2021;304: 114135.
5. Lafferty J, McCallum A, Pereira FCN. Conditional random fields: probabilistic models for segmenting and labeling sequence data. In: The eighteenth international conference on machine learning ICML, Williamstown. 2001. p. 282–9.
6. Hochreiter S, Schmidhuber J. Long short-term memory. Neural Comput. 1997;9(8):1735–80.
7. Vaswani A, Shazeer N, Parmar N, Uszkoreit J, Jones L, Gomez AN, Kaiser L. Attention is all you need. Adv Neural Inf Process Syst. 2017;30:50–4.
8. Kenton JDMWC, Toutanova LK. BERT: pre-training of deep bidirectional transformers for language understanding. In: Proceedings of NAACL-HLT. 2019. p. 4171–86.
9. Hendrycks D, Gimpel K. Bridging nonlinearities and stochastic regularizers with Gaussian error linear units. In: The 5th international conference on learning representation ICLR, Toulon. 2017. 213–126.

Chapter 3
Medical Named Entity Recognition Models with the Attention Distraction Mechanism

3.1 General Framework

In this chapter, a medical NER model, which is simply called as BERT-Attention-SCLSTM-CRF, is proposed by adding extended input units based on BiLSTM with attention distraction mechanism.

For the medical NER model, a parameter sharing unit is added to each LSTM neural unit on the basis of BiLSTM bidirectional network structure. Through using BiLSTM, the acquisition contextual relationship is further obtained, and the span of model learning context information is increased by using parameter sharing unit, and those further enhance the effect of entity recognition.

At present, LSTM is widely used in language generation, but LSTM has information loss due to the gradient when dealing with the long sequences of natural language tasks. To improve this problem, the coding model adds an extended parameter-sharing input unit compared with the traditional BiLSTM coding. The extended parameter sharing input unit improves the input gate of LSTM neural unit, which makes the neural network more suitable for the task of sequence labeling. The extended parameter sharing unit interacts the current information with the pre-and post-semantic representation information, and inputs this interaction information into the modified LSTM unit.

In addition, the BiLSTM model with extended input units designed in this chapter also uses the distraction mechanism to plan the relationship between texts so as to complete the entity recognition and classification in the sequence while ensuring the global information.

These above methods can improve the accuracy and stability of medical NER, and have better effect of entity boundary and classification. The medical NER model of BiLSTM with the extended input units is shown in Fig. 3.1.

S. Guo et al., *Clinical Chinese Named Entity Recognition in Natural Language Processing*, https://doi.org/10.1007/978-981-99-2665-7_3

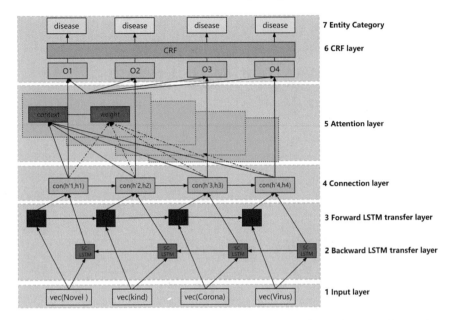

Fig. 3.1 The medical named entity recognition model of BiLSTM with the extended input units

3.2   Research Targeted Problem

Section 2.3.1 introduces the gradient problem of LSTM, but for the specific application of medical NER, LSTM faces capturing context information. Although LSTM's ability to obtain context dependencies is improved by comparing with RNN, LSTM is still unable to capture context information when the text length gradually increases, especially for CNER with long texts or long vocabularies, which weakens its ability to capture context information.

At present, some researches have shown that the problem of gradient and context information can be alleviated by using auxiliary information. Therefore, how to enhance the ability of LSTM to capture context information has become the focus of studies. The approach presented in this chapter is to control the flow of input context information by adding an additional input control unit.

3.3 Improved Neural Network Models

3.3.1 Extended Input Units

For proposing an extended input unit, the input of the neural network is received through the extended input module, and then connected with the input of LSTM through the output of the input unit. This way enhances the ability of the LSTM to control context semantics.

For constructing the extended input unit, the extended input module is divided into three parts such as the control gate operation, the shared unit operation and the output operation. For Fig. 3.2, r_t is the control gate operation, d_t is the shared unit operation, and W represents the weight of each gate, which is to be trained.

The control gate operation calculates the output of the preceding hidden layer together with the input of the preceding item, so that the control gate calculation includes the input and hidden information of the preceding moment. The control gate operation model of the extended input unit is Eq. 3.1.

$$r_t = \delta(W_{rx}[x_t, x_{t-1}] + \alpha W_{rh}h_{t-1}) \tag{3.1}$$

where δ is the ReLU function, i_t is the output of the extended input unit, also the input of the LSTM, W_{rx} is the weight of the dialogue extended input unit to the input x_t, W_{rh} is the weight of the dialogue expansion input unit to the hidden layer h_{t-1}, and W_{rx} and W_{rh} are parameters to be trained.

Fig. 3.2 LSTM neuron structure diagram with added the parameter sharing unit

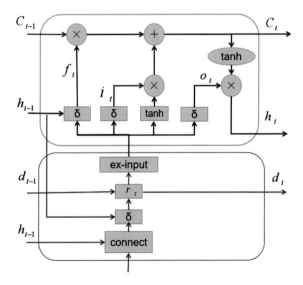

The initial implementation is that manipulating input accurately produces encoded input information, while at each time step, the shared unit determines the extent to which information should be retained for subsequent time steps.

Firstly, through model (3.1), r_t is obtained by calculating the input gate;

Secondly, the shared unit operation needs to be performed to obtain d_t, which is also the output of the dialogue extension input unit.

Thirdly, the sharing input unit can not only connect with LSTM, but also connect with other extended input units to share the parameter d_t and strengthen the control ability on semantic information.

The shared unit operation is Eq. 3.2:

$$d_t = r_t d_{t-1} \tag{3.2}$$

Finally, the final output i_t of the extended input unit through the dialogue is obtained, and its operation is Eq. 3.3:

$$
\begin{aligned}
i_t &= \tanh[W_{cd}(r_t * d_{t-1})] \\
&= \tanh\{W_{cd}[r_t * (\delta(W_{rx}x_t + W_{rh}h_{t-1})]\}
\end{aligned} \tag{3.3}
$$

where x_t is the input, h_{t-1} is the hidden layer, f_t is the forget gate, c_t is the memory unit, r_t is the control gate operation, d_t is the output of the shared unit, W_{rx} and W_{rh} are the weights to be trained for the extended input unit, and the parameter i_t is the output of the extended input unit, which also serves as the input of the LSTM.

According to the above presented model, the output of the parameter sharing unit is added as the input of the LSTM to form the LSTM neuron embedded in the parameter sharing unit. The presented neural network adopts the structure of BiLSTM, and adds an extended input unit and a hidden shared layer to improve the traditional BiLSTM's semantic information acquisition. On one hand, it can enhance the larger semantic information span of the model, and on the other hand, it can enrich the spatial semantic relation information by the interaction between the input and the current context.

The relational expression of the output operation unit is Eq. 3.4.

$$i_t^{SC} = 2\delta[(Q_t h_{t-2} i_{t-1})(R_t h_{t-1} i_{t-2})] \tag{3.4}$$

The memory unit of the LSTM neuron is realized by adding the output of the other layer of memory unit of BiLSTM to the input (seeing Fig. 3.2), so the relational expression of the LSTM neuron is Eq. 3.5:

$$
\begin{aligned}
f_t &= \delta(W_{fh}h_{t-1} + W_{fi}i_t^{sc}) \\
i_t &= \delta(W_{ih}h_{t-1} + W_{ix}i_t^{sc}) \\
o_t &= \delta(W_{oh}h_{t-1} + W_{ix}i_t^{sc}) \\
c_t' &= \tanh(W_{ch}h_{t-1} + W_{cx}i_t^{sc})
\end{aligned}
$$

$$c_t = f_t * c_{t-1} + i_t * c'_t$$
$$h_t = o_t * c_t$$
$$p_t = soft \max(h_t) \tag{3.5}$$

where h_{t-1} is the hidden layer, f_t is the forget gate, c'_t is the current input unit state, c_t is the memory unit, $W_{fh} W_{fi} W_{ix} W_{oh} W_{ch} W_{cx}$ are the weight of each gate, $*$ represents the Hadamard product, and i_t^{SC} is the output of the hidden shared layer obtained in Eq. 3.4, which is also the input of the LSTM.

3.3.2 Bi-SC-LSTM

After the SC-LSTM neural unit is constructed, the neural network is constructed according to the structure of two layers and two directions. The aim of double-layer is to model sentences bidirectionally by LSTM, and simultaneously to capture the information from back to front and from front to back. By inputting two-way information, BiLSTM-based learning model not only enriches the features of entities, but also improves the accuracy of entity classification. By using the two-way information, the hidden states of the first layer and the second layer will be updated according to the two-way hidden state of the previous moment, and specifically the parameter-sharing unit is obtained in a two-layer structure, so its hidden state is updated according to Eq. 3.7.

$$h_t = f(w_1 x_t + w_2 h_{t-1})$$
$$h'_t = f(w_3 x_t + w_4 h'_{t-1})$$
$$o_t = g(w_4 h_t + w_6 h'_t) \tag{3.7}$$

3.3.3 Attention Distraction Mechanisms

The encoder calculates the semantics of each word of the input sequence together, which results in the same semantics obtained by the decoder for all words, while cannot reflect the emphasis of the different input sequences. In order to solve semantic invisibility, by adopting the attention distraction mechanism, the different positions of the input sequence have different effects on each output of the decoder, so each output of the decoder should be computed to get different semantics. The flow chart of the attention distraction mechanism is shown in Fig. 3.3.

First, the forward context vector o_t^1 and the backward context vector o_t^2, which are generated by the BiLSTM model after adding the expanded input unit, are connected by the fully connected layer. BiLSTMs can capture the semantics of the forward and

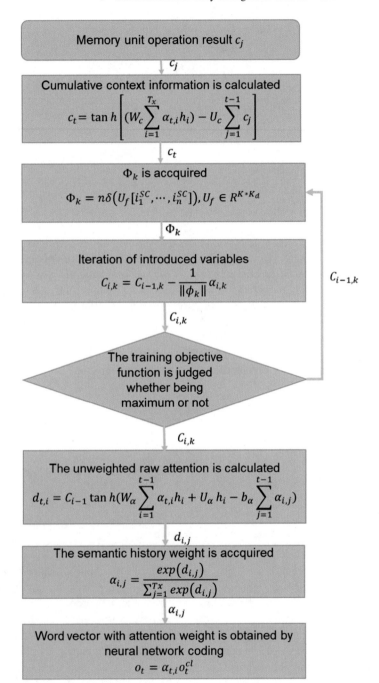

Fig. 3.3 Flow chart of attention distraction mechanism

backward phases. The BiLSTM model after adding the extended input unit has two layers of LSTM, a forward LSTM and a backward LSTM. For each token, the forward LSTM processes the vector o_t^1 which is used to calculate the forward context vector representation from scratch and vice versa, the Backward LSTM, from which to process the end of the sentence, calculates the backward context vector representing o_t^2. The forward and backward vectors represent the connection of o_t^1 and o_t^2, and take the semantic representation LSTM layer to connect to form the final word vector o_t.

o_t is obtained after passing through the connection layer with

$$o_t = o_t^2 \oplus o_t^1 = [o_t^2, o_t^1].$$

where $\oplus$ represents the direct sum, $u \oplus v = [u_1 \ldots u_r, v_1 \ldots v_r]^T$ for any vectors $u = [u_1 \ldots u_r]^T$, $v = [v_1 \ldots v_r]$ in r-dimensional space.

The calculation model of the connection layer is Eq. 3.8,

$$v_a = \tanh[\omega_1 o_t^1 \cdot o_t^2 + \omega_2 (o_t^1 \oplus o_t^2)] \tag{3.8}$$

where v_a represents the bidirectional context vector, and ω_1, ω_2 are weight parameters.

The accumulated context information and the depenalized context information are used to compute the next context information, and the context semantic information contains the hidden semantic information in the statement, so it is necessary to use the results of the hidden layer and the memory unit in the neural network.

The model c_t for calculating contextual semantic information is Eq. 3.9.

$$c_t = \tanh\left[\left(W_c \sum_{i=1}^{Tx} \alpha_{t,i} h_i\right) - U_c \sum_{j=1}^{t-1} c_j\right] \tag{3.9}$$

where h_i is the output of the hidden layer, c_i is the cumulative sum of the output of the memory unit, W_c and U_c are set as the diagonal matrices with the parameters to be learned, $\alpha_{t,i}$ is the attention weight applied to the decoding time t, and $\tanh$ denotes a hyperbolic function.

By using the original attention without the weight of historical attention, the semantic weight of historical attention $\alpha_{i,j}$ is obtained, whose calculation model is Eq. 3.10.

$$\alpha_{t,i} = \frac{\exp\left(C_{i-1,k} v_a^T \tanh\left(W_a \sum_{i=1}^{t-1} \alpha_{t,i}' h_i + U_a h_i - b_a \sum_{j=1}^{t-1} \alpha_{i,j}'\right)\right)}{\sum_{j=1}^{Tx} \exp\left(C_{j-1,k} v_a^T \tanh\left(W_a \sum_{i=1}^{t-1} \alpha_{t,j}' h_j + U_a h_j - b_a \sum_{j=1}^{t-1} \alpha_{j,j}'\right)\right)} \tag{3.10}$$

where v_a represents the bidirectional context vector obtained after passing through the connection layer in Eq. 3.8, and $C_{i-1,k}$ denotes to get the expression of sentence structure information that a word has to generate information from Eq. 3.11.

For the attention distraction mechanism by introducing a variable $C_{i,k}$ in Eq. 3.10, the difference from other attention mechanisms lies in the distraction effect of the variable $C_{i,k}$. That is to say, $C_{i,k}$ is used to indicate how much sentence structure information is generated for a word, and how much sentence structure information is not generated.

The value of $C_{i,k}$ optimizes the attention coefficient so that the attention distraction mechanism can contain semantic information and simultaneously prevent iterative process overfitting. The iterative model of $C_{i,k}$ is Eq. 3.11.

$$C_{i,k} = a_t \left(C_{i-1,k} - \frac{1}{\|\phi_k\|} \alpha_{i,k} \right) \tag{3.11}$$

where a_t is a random discarding coefficient, obeying to Bernoulli distribution, $a_{i,k}$ is divided by any ϕ_k value, so that the value of each reduction of topic words with a large amount of information is correspondingly smaller, which ensures that the final generated information can be more. n is the text length input to the neural network, i_t^{SC} is each word input to the neural network, U_f is the parameter of the generation training, and δ is the ReLU function.

The calculation model of ϕ_k is Eq. 3.12:

$$\phi_k = n\delta \left(U_f \left[i_1^{SC}, \ldots, i_n^{SC} \right] \right), U_f \in R^{K^* K_d} \tag{3.12}$$

Finally, when the training objective function reaches the optimization, the training parameters of the model are obtained, and simultaneously the updated iteration for C_i stops, thus the training objective function is obtained.

Here k is the number of words, the h_i^1 of the model is the ith hidden state of the first layer of the encoding, and h_i^2 is the hidden state of the jth input of the encoding.

The vector set is represented by T_i, which is calculated as Eq. 3.13.

$$T_i = \sum_{j=1}^{k} \alpha_{t,j} h_j \tag{3.13}$$

where P is the probability distribution of each word, and c_t is the obtained contextual semantic information.

The model for calculating P is Eq. 3.14.

$$P\left(y \middle| y_{i-1}, h_i^1, T_i \right) = soft \max \left(g \left(h_i^1 \right) \right) \tag{3.14}$$

where $g(.)$ denotes the degree of relationship between hidden information and output information, which calculation model is Eq. 3.15.

$$g(h, y_{t-1}, c_t) = W_0 \tanh(N y_{t-1} + C_0 c_t + U_h h_t) \tag{3.15}$$

where h_i^1 is the hidden layer of LSTM, y_t is the output of LSTM at time t, the hidden layer $f(\cdot)$ is defined in Eq. 3.5, and the calculation model of h_i^1 is Eq. 3.16.

$$h_i^1 = f\left(h_{i-1}^1, y_{i-1}, T_i\right) \tag{3.16}$$

The training objective function is Eq. 3.17.

$$\left(\theta^*, \eta^*\right) = \arg\max_{\theta, \eta} \sum_{n=1}^{N} \left\{ \log P(y_n | x_n; \theta, \eta) - \lambda \left\{ \sum_{k=1}^{K} \left(\|\phi_k\| - \sum_{i=1}^{I} \alpha_{i,k} \right)^2 \right\} \right\} \tag{3.17}$$

where θ, η are the training parameter sets in the above steps,

$$\theta = \left\{ W_{rx}, W_{rh}, W_{fh}, W_{ih}, W_{ft}, W_{ix}, W_{cx}, W_{ch}, W_c, W_a \right\},$$
$$\eta = \left\{ U_c, U_a, b_a, U_f, W_0, C_0, U_h \right\}$$

After the neural network model is built and the objective function is determined, the training process is carried out by the above optimization algorithm.

3.3.4 Decoding Layer

NER is essentially a sequence labeling task, and since labels are not independent on each other, it is necessary to thoroughly understand the internal relationship of labels based on the label dataset. As a conditional probability model, CRF can deal with contextual feature information and effectively consider constraints among labels to reduce illogical sequences. In addition, CRF is globally normalized on the basis of maximum entropy Markov wandering, which can observe not only single observation state, but also sequence length, context word and so on. The problem of standard bias is solved by enumerating the possibilities of all output sequences. Finally, the Viterbi algorithm is used to find the optimal path to reach the maximum probability in the prediction process.

The CRF [1] model uses the regularized maximum similarity estimation to maximize the probability, and the gradient descent optimization algorithm is adopted. The maximum likelihood function of CRF model is Eq. 3.18.

$$\log(p(Y|S)) = s(X, Y) - \log\left(\sum_{Y_i \in Y_A} e^{s(X, Y_i)} \right) \tag{3.18}$$

3.4   Experiments and Simulation Results

3.4.1   Datasets

In order to prove the superiority of the proposed method to the traditional model, the proposed method and the related baseline model are trained and evaluated based on the 2019 CCKS dataset. In the 2019 CCKS-CNER dataset, there are six categories of clinical entities to be identified, including diseases, image examination, test, treatment, drugs, and anatomy. Each type of entity is shown in Fig. 3.4 and Table 3.1, respectively.

Where Entities in the Chinese text are represented by "BIO", where "B", "I" and "O" represent the beginning of the entity, the Chinese characters inside the entity, and other unrelated characters, respectively.

Fig. 3.4 The number of entities in the training data

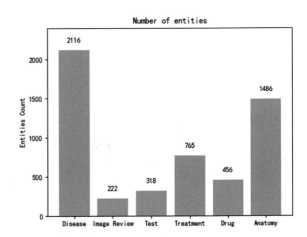

Table 3.1 The number of entities in the training data

Entity categories	Number
Diseases	2116
Image review	222
Test	318
Treatment	765
Drug	456
Body parts	1486
Total	5363

3.4.2 Experiments

The input model adopts the pretraining BERT model to dynamically embed GloVe's static word embedding. A BERT model is a typical representation learning, which is pretrained on a large unlabeled text corpus to learn better text features. BERT is often applied to a wide range of tasks through fine-tuning. Therefore, the BERT model is used to transform the text into embedded text and capture deep knowledge of the text, including parts of speech, implicit language rules, and main sentence features.

The model is trained with a batch size 50 and a learning rate 0.001. The 300-dimensional word vectors used in the experiment are a pretrained GloVe word vectors based on a large number of clinical medical records and template image description texts.

Adam [2] is selected as the optimization algorithm with the regularization parameter 1e−10 and an epoch 50.

Gated recurrent unit (GRU) is also trained and tested in the comparison model. GRU is a variant of LSTM, which simplifies the structure of LSTM and further alleviates the long dependence. By integrating the gate control units and adding updated units, the number of parameters in the neural network is reduced. In the case of lack of training data, GRU may speed up its training speed, and easier to achieve generalization than LSTM, but its flexibility is insufficient.

3.4.3 Introduction to Comparison Models

The contrast models of CRF, LSTM-CRF, GRU-CRF, SCLSTM-CRF, BERT-CRF, BERT-LSTM-CRF are selected. The models have the same parameters as BERT-SCLSTM-CRF in terms of embedding, optimization algorithm, learning rate and dimension of hidden layer.

3.4.4 Experimental Results

A performance comparison for NER for Each Models is shown as Table 3.2.

In Table 3.2, two embedding methods are adopted, one is static embedding (e. g. GloVe) and the other is dynamic embedding (BERT embedding). Based on these, it can be seen that the SCLSTM proposed in this chapter in both GloVe and Bert embedding are higher than other models, F_1 scores reach to 0.82 and 0.87 respectively. For GloVe embedding, the F_1 score of SCLSTM is 1–2% higher than that of other models, and for Bert embedding, the F_1 score of SCLSTM is 2–3% higher than that of other models.

Table 3.2 A performance comparison for named entity recognition for each models

Methods	Precision	Recall	F1
GloVe-CRF	0.75	0.73	0.74
GloVe-LSTM-CRF	0.79	0.81	0.80
GloVe-GRU-CRF	0.80	0.80	0.81
GloVe-SCLSTM-CRF	0.80	0.81	0.82
BERT-CRF	0.83	0.801	0.82
BERT-LSTM-CRF	0.86	0.91	0.85
BERT-GRU-CRF	0.85	0.86	0.85
BERT-SCLSTM-CRF	0.83	0.84	0.84
BERT-Attention-SCLSTM-CRF	0.87	0.88	0.87

3.4.5 Experiment Analysis

According to the experimental results, SCLSTM has more advantages in medical NER, and LSTM can acquire longer context-dependence by adding parameter sharing unit, especially in the recognition of medical entities.

In Table 3.2, SCLSTM-CRF achieves an F_1 score of 82%, while the F_1 score of LSTM-CRF is 80%. For BERT embedding, SCLSTM-CRF achieves an F_1-score of 87%, and LSTM-CRF achieves an F_1-score of 85%.

The reasons why the performance of F_1 can be improved are as follows. On one hand, SCLSTM is more suitable for recognizing longer medical terms, for example, internal fixation of left rib fracture, arteriovenous bypass for renal dialysis in left forearm, left thyroid adenoma resection and other longer terms, can achieve a higher accuracy. On the other hand, due to the establishment of the attention distraction mechanism, the relationship among words in different positions can be learned in the entire text segment, and SCLSTM can acquire longer context dependencies, thereby can easily acquire context dependencies in more longer terms and longer texts in clinical medicine.

3.5 Conclusions

In this chapter, a neural network model is proposed, which utilizes an LSTM with augmented input units combined with a distraction mechanism. In the neural network structure, the extended input unit is combined with the LSTM neural unit, and the improved LSTM neural unit is formed according to the double-layer bidirectional structure to form the SC-BiLSTM neural network model.

For the NER task, the proposed SCLSTM model in this chapter acts as the encoder and CRF does as the decoder, so the above encoder-decoder can effectively obtain the entity information of the sequence annotation of the text.

For the presented model, the parameter sharing unit is used to enhance the ability of obtaining context information, which broadens the maximum boundary of LSTM. In order to verify the validity and superiority of the presented model, the data set of 2019 CCKS is used to train and test the presented model, and the experimental results show that the accuracy, recall and F1 score of the presented model are higher than those of other contrast models.

References

1. Lafferty J, McCallum A, Pereira FCN. Conditional random fields: probabilistic models for segmenting and labeling sequence data. In: The eighteenth international conference on machine learning ICML, Williamstown. 2001. p. 282–9.
2. Kingma DP, Ba J. Adam: a method for stochastic optimization. In: The 3rd international conference on learning representations ICLR (poster), San Diego. 2015.

Chapter 4
Transformer Entity Automatic Extraction Models in Multi-layer Soft Location Matching Format

4.1 General Framework

In this chapter, a multi-layer soft position matching format Transformer method is proposed to extract clinical medical entities. The new model is shown in Fig. 4.1. The proposed model consists of five parts: WordPiece preprocessing module, BERT module, multi-layer soft position matching module, word format Transformer, and fuzzy CRF module.

Firstly, WordPiece preprocessing module is used to preprocess the data to segment the vocabulary to obtain a dictionary. Secondly, the BERT module is used to preprocess the input data to obtain the underlying features of the input text, such as parts of speech and features of the character. And simultaneously the MLM required for BERT pre-training, a dynamic adaptive masking strategy is adopted to learn more sufficient contextual information on the basis of bidirectional learning. Thirdly, the multi-layer soft position matching module is used to select the word segmentation results. Fourthly, the selected word segmentation results are input into the word format Transformer module, word and word order information is used to introduce vocabulary information to the greatest extent without loss. Finally, the fuzzy CRF layer decodes the output of the previous module into the optimal sequence and outputs the annotation information.

4.2 Research Targeted Problem

The NER is a key and fundamental part of many NLP tasks, including knowledge mapping, question answering system and machine translation. When extracting entities from EHRs, NER models predominantly employ LSTM and have achieved a striking performance in clinical NER. However, these LSTM-based models often need to increase the depth of the network to capture long-distance dependencies. Because of this, these LSTM-based models achieve high accuracy, and often require

© The Author(s), under exclusive license to Springer Nature Singapore Pte Ltd. 2023   45
S. Guo et al., *Clinical Chinese Named Entity Recognition in Natural Language Processing*, https://doi.org/10.1007/978-981-99-2665-7_4

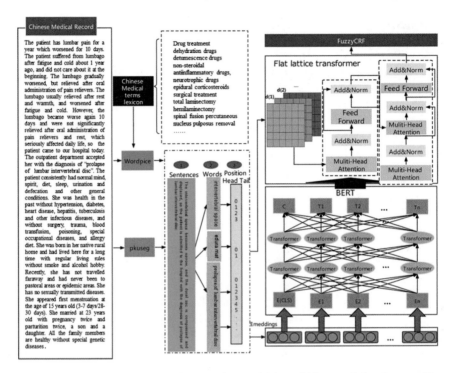

Fig. 4.1 Transformer entity automatic extraction model in multi-layer soft location matching format

long training times and large amounts of training data, which hinders the adoption of LSTM-based models in clinical scenarios with the limited training time. Therefore, modelling, which can capture the contextual information and simultaneously realize parallel computing in less computing time, has already become a key issue. Therefore, inspired by the Transformer, combining the Transformer with lattice Chinese word information can form a FLAT, which can have long-distance dependencies like the LSTM.

4.3 Multilayer Soft Position Matching Format Transformer

4.3.1 WordPiece Word Segmentation

Since the smallest unit of Chinese is Chinese characters, Chinese sentences cannot be split into letters like English, so a WordPiece is not suitable for Chinese. However, the extensive length of the terms used in the field of clinical medicine makes the Word-Piece appropriate for the field of clinical medicine. The WordPiece has a stronger guarantee that each subword unit has been presented in the training text. It enables the model to try to learn the representations of words from a vocabulary. The main implementation of WordPiece is the BPE (Byte Pair Encoding) algorithm. The WordPiece is essentially a data-driven approach [1]. For a given constantly changed vocabulary, it selects adjacent subwords that maximize the probability, the language model will be added to the list of words, and merges the selected adjacent subwords into new subwords.

First, the WordPieces algorithm is needed to confirm the training corpus, and D is used to indicate the desired number of tokens. The goal of the optimization is to choose the WordPieces to minimize the number of the WordPieces in the resulting vocabulary when subwords are obtained according to the chosen WordPiece model. Biomedical domain texts contain a large number of domain-specific proper nouns (e.g. BRCA1, c.248T>C etc.) and proprietary terms (e.g. transcription, antimicrobials etc.), therefore BERT needs to be pre-trained to learn preliminary medical domain text information form the BioBERT.

For the tokenization, the BioBERT uses the WordPiece tokenization, which alleviates the problem of semantic inadequacy. With the WordPiece tokenization, any new words can be represented by frequent subwords (such as immunoglobulins), and better performance can be achieved in downstream tasks with lattice terms. But for Chinese language, there is no WordPiece segmentation methods, because the smallest unit of Chinese is a word, and it cannot be divided into a combination of letters like English.

However, because of the larger length of terms in the field of clinical medicine, a WordPiece is more suitable for the field of clinical medicine. An example of this is shown in Table 4.1.

For example, "oxaliper (奥沙利珀)" or "oxaliper (奥沙利柏)", brain craniotomy, left frontal lobe glioma resection and frontal lobe lesion resection, etc. The WordPiece splits the entire word to preprocess a given piece of data. It is implemented by using the double-byte Encoding (Byte-Pair Encoding, BPE). This section uses the WordPiece to form a new vocabulary based on the original vocabulary, and provides supports for the subsequent word segmentation based on this vocabulary. The WordPieces can realize the flexibility of Chinese characters in medical records. The WordPiece is used to process the Chinese medical terms in Table 4.1, and obtained a dictionary that contains frequently appearing subwords in Table 4.1. This obtained dictionary is the basis and premise of the word mesh Transformer in Sect. 4.5.

4.3.2 BERT

4.3.2.1 The BERT Structure

The BERT model is often used as the backbone, which is obtained through pre training of Chinese clinical texts, and adds several Chinese clinical commonly used texts that have not been included before. So that the model can adapt to downstream biomedical text mining tasks and is pretrained through the clinical texts. When the

Table 4.1 Partial glossary of longer Chinese medical terms

Glossary 1	Glossary 2
胸腔镜胸腺囊肿切除术 (Thoracoscopic thymectomy)	胸腺病损切除术 (Excision of lesion of thymus/thymectomy)
耻骨上经膀胱前列腺剜除术 (Suprapubic transvesical enucleation of prostate)	耻骨上经膀胱前列腺切除术 (Suprapubic transvesical prostatectomy/TVP/SPPC/)
左眼眶减压术 (Decompression of left orbit)	眶减压术 (Orbital decompression)
右脑室-腹腔分流术 (Right ventriculo-peritoneal shunt/ventriculoperitoneal shunt/V-P shunt)	侧脑室腹腔内分流术 (Lateral ventriculoperitoneal shunt)
开放膀胱切开取石术 (Open cystotomy for lithotomy)	膀胱切开取石术 (Cystolithotomy/cystotomy and lithotomy)
股骨胫骨折空心钉内固定术 (Internal fixation of femoral and tibial fractures with cannulated nails)	股骨内固定术 (Internal fixation of femur)
左侧肋骨骨折内固定术 (Internal fixation of left rib fracture)	肋骨内固定术 (Internal fixation of rib)
左前臂为肾透析的动静脉人工血管搭桥术 (Arteriovenous bypass graft for renal dialysis with left forearm)	为肾透析, 动静脉吻合术 (Arteriovenous anastomosis for renal dialysis)
左甲状腺腺瘤摘除术 (Excision of left thyroid adenoma)	甲状腺病损切除术 (Excision of lesion of thyroid)
显微镜下经蝶垂体瘤切除术 (Transsphenoidal microsurgery for pituitary adenoma)	经蝶骨垂体病损切除术 (Transsphenoidal pituitary lesion resection)
胸腔镜下右上肺叶切除术 (Thoracoscopic right upper lobectomy)	胸腔镜下肺叶切除术 (Thoracoscopic lobectomy of lung)
VATS 左后纵隔肿物切除术 (VATS left posterior mediastinal mass resection)	胸腔镜下纵隔病损切除术 (Thoracoscopic mediastinal lesion resection)
腰 1-2 椎管内占位切除术 (Space occupying resection of lumbar 1-2 spinal canal)	脊髓或脊膜病损的切除术或破坏术 (Excision/destruction of spinal cord/meningeal lesions)
全部膝关节置换 (施乐辉) (Total knee replacement (Smith & Nephew))	全部膝关节置换 (Total knee replacement)
膀胱镜活检术 (Cystoscopy biopsy)	闭合性 [经尿道] 膀胱活组织检查 (Closed [transurethral] bladder biopsy)
甲状腺右叶腺叶切除术 (Adenectomy of right lobe of thyroid)	单侧甲状腺叶切除术 (Unilateral lobectomy of thyroid)

(continued)

Table 4.1 (continued)

Glossary 1	Glossary 2
子宫下段剖宫产术 + 臀牵引术 (Cesarean section of lower segment of uterus + hip traction)	低位子宫下段剖宫产 ## 臀位牵引 (Low uterine lower segment cesarean section ## breech traction)
左侧颅骨钻孔慢性硬膜下血肿冲洗引流术 (Irrigation and drainage of chronic subdural hematoma drilled in the left skull)	颅骨钻孔引流术 (Cranial trepanation and drainage)
右额钻孔硬脑膜下血肿引流术 (Drainage of subdural hematoma by right frontal trepanation)	脑膜切开术 (Incision of cerebral meninges)

model performs the NER task, the model itself can contain the information of multiple domain specific nouns in the biomedical corpus, so as to better complete the NER task.

As shown in Fig. 4.2, the BERT has a simple architecture based on bidirectional transformers, which uses a single output layer to calculate the label's probability based on the representation from its last layer. However, the BioBERT can directly learn word embedding during pretraining and fine-tuning. The BERT is generally set up by a 12-layer bidirectional transformer, which simultaneously draws on the self attention mechanism and the residual mechanism of CNN, so the BERT model has fast training speeds and the strong expression ability. It needs to point out that the RNN loop structure is also abandoned. In order to apply to various downstream text mining tasks, especially the NER, the BioBERT is firstly fine tuned, which is mainly to modify the architecture with a smile. The BioBERT's NER has been fine-tuned based on the following representative biomedical text mining tasks.

The BERT is an unsupervised depth bidirectional language representation model for pre-training. In order to accurately represent the context-related semantic information in the EMR, it is necessary to mobilize the interface of the model to obtain the

Fig. 4.2 Partial transformer decoding diagram

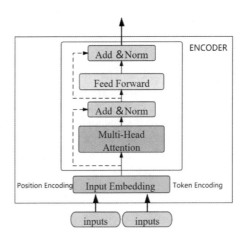

embedded representation of each word in the EMR. The BERT uses a deep two-way transformer encoder as the main structure of the model. As shown in Fig. 4.2, the Transformer introduces the self-attention mechanism and also draws on the residual mechanism of the CNN, so the model training speed is fast and the expression ability is strong. It also abandons the RNN loop structure. The Transformer performs self-attention on the sequence through H attention heads respectively, and then concatenates the results of the H heads. For simplicity, the head index is ignored in the following model. The result of each self-attention is calculated as Eqs. 4.1 and 4.2.

$$Attention(Q, K, V) = soft \max\left(\frac{QK^T}{\sqrt{d_k}}\right)V \tag{4.1}$$

$$[Q, K, V] = E_x[W_q, W_k, W_v] \tag{4.2}$$

where d_k is the dimension of each head, that is, the dimension of K of each attention head. E_x is token embedding. $W_q W_k W_v$ are the parameters to be learned.

It is pointed out that the English model in the original BERT, which uses the addition of three types of word vectors (e.g. word embedding, phrases embedding, and position embedding), finally enters the input vectors of BERT, while the Chinese model does not have the operation of word segmentation, without word embedding, only using word vectors and position vectors.

The general classification task of training language model uses the final hidden state of the first CLS token to predict. Most of common fine-tuning uses this method. Of course, it can be modified to obtain all parameters of the last layer for a max pooling operation. As shown in Fig. 4.3, for sequence labeling, the token representations are fed to the output layer for token-level tasks such as sequence labeling. CLS and SEP are the necessary tokens for BERT data organization. To enable the BERT to process various downstream tasks, the input of the BERT can represent a single sentence or a pair of sentences for a token sequence.

4.3.2.2 Masking Language Modelling

The random masking strategy is mainly used to represent the model to learn deep bidirectional representation information. The strategy is to cover a certain proportion of the input simply and randomly, and complete the pretraining by predicting the masked words. This process is called masking language models (MLM).

In this case, as in standard language models, the final hidden vector corresponding to the mask token is fed into the output softmax on the vocabulary where the best prediction is obtained. The objective function of a MLM is to predict the cross-entropy loss of mask tokens.

The MLM randomly blocks 15% of the words at each iteration. The goal of the model is to predict these words based on the context. The MLM is very suitable for long sequence text NER tasks by simultaneously using a converter encoder with

Fig. 4.3 BERT fine-tuning on NER task

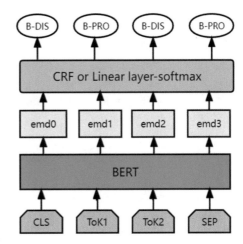

strong extraction capability and a two-way training form. So the MLM is very suitable for long-sequence text NER tasks (Table 4.2).

Assuming that the original sequence is $x = [x_1, x_j, \ldots, x_T]$ and $x \backslash \{x_i\}$ represents the sequence after replacing the ith token or vocabulary with the mask token, the MLM model is modeled as follows:

$$p(x_i, x_j, x_k, \ldots | x \backslash \{x_i, x_j, x_k, \ldots\}) \tag{4.3}$$

Table 4.2 Comparison of masking strategies

Masking strategy	Content	Specific method
Static masking strategy	The original BERT model will extract 15% of the tokens in the training task for mask, but the mask will not change in each epoch later, which will lead to no change in the mask during the whole pre training process, that is, it is a single static mask	In creating pre-training data, the data is masked in advance. To make full use of the data, dupe_Factor is defined, which can be copied into the dupe_Factor copies, and then the same data can have different masks. Note that not all of these data are fed to the same epoch, but to different epochs. For example, dupe_Factor = 10, epoch = 40 means that each mask method will be used 4 times in training
Dynamic masking strategy	Each time the training example is fed to the model, the random mask is performed. That is, the mask is dynamically generated at each time and the data is input to the model	10 copies of the original corpus are copied. For each corpus, 15% of the tokens are randomly selected to cover, replace and maintain
Span masking strategy	Covering the whole word directly	Randomly covering a continuous paragraph of words

Assuming that only one token is masked at each time, the distribution of the model is as follows:

$$p(x_i|x\backslash\{x_i\}), i = 1, 2, 3, \ldots, T \tag{4.4}$$

The goal of the MLM is that a single model can simultaneously obtain the prediction of each mask as model 4.5 in each training.

$$p(x_T|x\backslash\{x_T\}), T = 1, 2, 3, \ldots, n \tag{4.5}$$

So, that is to say, when $p(x_i|x\backslash\{x_i\})$ is modeled, it means that the ith output does not always contain the token information of the ith token. In order to ensure that $p(x_i|x\backslash\{x_i\})$ does not contain token information, the neural network is presented to $p(x_i|x\backslash\{x_i\})$ and then combines the original character features as the final feature identifier, as shown in Eq. 4.6.

$$e'_i = p(x_i|x\backslash\{x_i\})e_m + (1 - p(x_i|x\backslash\{x_i\}))e_i \tag{4.6}$$

4.3.2.3   Next Sentence Prediction (NSP)

The pretraining BERT is realized by an unsupervised learning, which obtains text information through a large amount of unsupervised data. After pretraining, most of the BERT parameters have been trained. When applying to downstream tasks, only a few rounds of supervised learning on the dataset are required to complete the task with high performances.

For the pretraining task of sentence continuous prediction, the input of BERT can be any span of continuous text, and it is not required to follow the sentence in real life, but the token sequence is accepted by the real BERT. Therefore, the BERT can connect two sentences together and then process them, and Token sequences are created by combining the WordPiece embedding with 30,000 token vocabularies.

For example, in pretraining NSP, the first marker [CLS] of each sequence is a special classification token, whose role is to fuse two sequences together to form a new single sequence. Two ways are used to distinguish sentences such that a special token [SEP] is used to separate them, and/or learning embedment is added to each tag to indicate whether it is continuous.

The NSP aims to train the model to infer the relationship between two sentences and obtain sentence level text features. That is, two sentences A and B are given, and B has a half probability of being the next sentence of A, the training model is used to predict whether B is the next sentence of A, and the crossed entropy loss function is adapted during the training. In Fig. 4.3, the sentences are separated by CLS and SEP.

This research is to train and complete the BERT model on the Chinese clinical text corpus, and simultaneously uses the covering method of the Whole Entity Masking

(WEM) and the Whole Span Masking to cover medical entities and synonyms similar to this medical Entity, explicitly injects this medical knowledge into the BERT model, then uses the model parameters of the BERT-base for initialization, and finally completes the pretraining.

The simplified and main steps of the WEM are as follows:

(1) The medical entities are identified and predicted by using NER;
(2) The medical entities is post-processed by using Chinese medical knowledge atlas.

The simplified and main steps of the WSM are as follows:

(1) The phrases are extracted through using the Auto-phrase;
(2) The common medical phrases are retrieved from the Alibaba Cognitive Concept Atlas;
(3) A binary classifier is trained to classify the medical extracted phrases with the Auto-phrases.

4.4 The Lattice Transformer

4.4.1 The General

The Transformer mainly uses the self-attention mechanism to get the context dependent on the information of the sequence, and calculates the attention scores between two words in different positions, and then models the dependency relationship in the sequence. Since the self-attention does not learn the distance among words in the sequence, the time complexity of the self-attention will not increase with the longer distance. Because of these factors, the Transformer is still unable to achieve the performance of the LSTM in some tasks that need to focus on the location information, such as the NER, the QA dialogue, etc. Therefore, strengthening the Transformer's position awareness and context dependencies has become the main purpose of the word lattice Transformer.

4.4.2 The Word Lattice Structure Transformer

This section proposes the construction of the word lattice structure Transformer model [2]. First, the Chinese texts are segmented, and then a lattice structure is formed according to the segmentation result, and then the lattice results are flattened by the same head and tail method as the FLAT [3], which is convenient for the input to the Transformer. The obtained word lattice structure makes the interaction between the characters and the lexical information more direct, and the Transformer establishes the long-term dependencies of the sequence. How to select and integrate the characters and the vocabularies based on the sequence annotation has always been the research content of CNER.

The adoption of Chinese lattice structure can not only alleviate the sparsity and fuzziness of Chinese vocabularies, but also introduce word segmentation information into the model to achieve high performances. In addition, it provides rich entity boundary information for NER tasks.

The lattice-structured Transformer alleviates the BERT's inability to obtain dependencies among mask positions and the need for extensive computation to predict mask words. In this section, the matrix lattice is obtained by splitting sentences according to the dictionary in the WordPiece Sect. 4.3. For the flattened lattice structure, the span in the plane grid has the head and tail of sub-words in the thesaurus, as shown in Fig. 4.4, which can strengthen the entity boundary. For span position coding, the absolute position coding is abandoned, and the relative position coding is correspondingly adapted to construct head positions coding and tail positions coding, as shown in Fig. 4.5. According to the above designed position encoding, the relative position coding of span introduces vocabulary information into the Transformer without loss. Therefore, the lattice-structured Transformer can make full use of the lattice information and improve the performance of CNER. The word lattice structure Transformer encoder needs the span of Chinese words with different lengths to encode the interactions in these words. In order to enable the Transformer to obtain the location information, the traditional location embedding mostly adopts the method of absolute location embedding.

Since the Transformer input is the addition of word vector and position encoding, the dimensions of the two should be the same.

When the Transformer position is embedded, it uses different periodic functions such as sine and/or cosine functions with different frequencies to map the position. The mapping relationship is Eq. 4.7

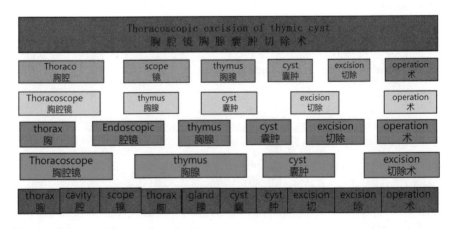

Fig. 4.4 Schematic diagram of word grid structure

Fig. 4.5 Structure of the flat word lattice transformer (FLAT)

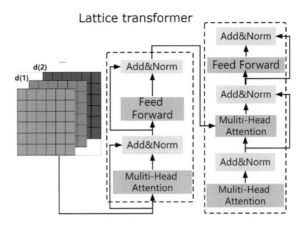

$$PE_{(pos,2i)} = \sin\left(p/10{,}000^{2i/d_{model}}\right)$$
$$PE_{(pos,2i+1)} = \cos\left(p/10{,}000^{2i/d_{model}}\right) \tag{4.7}$$

where p is the position and i is the dimension. The sine and cosine functions make each dimension of position coding correspond to a trigonometric function value, whose wavelengths form a geometric series from 2π to $10{,}000 \cdot 2\pi$. The sine and cosine functions are guaranteed to have the same positional embedding in each step, and the sine and cosine functions as periodic functions can satisfy this mapping condition as well. The above embedding allows the model to easily learn relative positions. The sine and cosine functions ensure that for any fixed offset, PE_{p+k} can be expressed as PE_p, then the position embedding PE_p is added to the word embedding to complete the embedding of the Transformer. And this word embedding method leads to the loss of performance, and the location information will be lost with the training of the model. Therefore, the dynamic relative position embedding becomes a position embedding method to avoid the Transformer position loss.

The relative position embedding injects the same information into the attention score of each layer, rather than adding some biases to the initial embedding statically. In order to avoid the performance degrading in long sequences caused by absolute position embedding, more importantly, the relative position embedding is more suitable for the time biased sequence information, which is more intuitive and universal.

For the standard Transformer, the attention score between query q_i and key vector k_j within the same segment can be decomposed into Eq. 4.8:

$$A_{i,j}^{abs} = E_{x_i}^T W_q^T W_k E_{x_j} + E_{x_i}^T W_q^T W_k U_j$$
$$+ U_i^T W_q^T W_k E_{x_j} + U_i^T W_q^T W_k U_j \tag{4.8}$$

While using the relative position encoding, the corresponding model becomes Eq. 4.9.

$$A_{i,j}^{rel} = E_{x_i}^T W_q^T W_{k,E} E_{x_j} + E_{x_i}^T W_q^T W_{k,r} R_{i-j}$$
$$+ u^T W_k E_{x_j} + u^T W_k R_{i-j} \qquad (4.9)$$

According to the relative distance between each key vector k_j and its own q_j, i.e. $i - j$, the above input position information can be guaranteed.

In fact, a set of relative position codes $R \in R^{L_{max} \times d}$ can be created, where the i-th row R_i represents the relative distance i between two positions. By dynamically injecting relative distances into the attention scores, the query vector can easily distinguish the representations of $x_{\tau,j}$ and $x_{\tau+1,j}$ from their different distances, and make the state reused mechanism feasible. And simultaneously, any temporal information does not lose because absolute positions can be recursively recovered from relative distances.

Compared with the two models, all occurrences of absolute position embedding U_j are replaced by their corresponding counterparts R_{i-j}; Moreover, a trainable parameter u^T is introduced to replace the query U_i^T in the Eq. 4.9. In this case, since the query vectors of all query locations are the same, the attention bias for different words should remain unchanged regardless of the query location.

In addition, the two weight matrices $W_{k,E}$ and $W_{k,r}$ are separated to generate content-based key vectors and location-based key vectors respectively. The relative position embedding includes the interactions among the input and the input, the input and the position, the position and the input, and the position and the position. These four interactions overlap to a certain extent. The current relative position embedding method minimizes overlapping delivery relationships by retaining at least an interaction and no more than three interactions, such that T5 [1] only retains three interactions.

Therefore, the goal of this model is to use the Transformer of the Chinese character lattice to further reduce the overlapping interaction between the position and the input, and the relative position embedding is Eq. 4.10 [1].

$$A_{i,j}^{rel} = E_{x_i}^T W_k^T W_q E_{x_i} + E_{x_i}^T W_k^T W_q R_{i,j} + R_{i,j}^T W_k^T W_q E_{x_i} \qquad (4.10)$$

In order to encode the position of the span in the lattice structure, the position encoding methods, which can be applicable to the standard Transformer, is not directly adopted, but the relative position embedding of the span information [2] is added to achieve the modeling of the position encoding and position difference of the span.

For the segmentation of word lattice structure, using WordPiece to segment Chinese words is firstly proposed in this chapter. As shown in Fig. 4.5, the input of the FLAT model is a sequence of characters and/or all subsequences of characters matching with dictionary D, which is modeled with using a large amount of raw texts in Sect. 4.3. Here D is a dictionary obtained by using WordPiece automatically segmenting large raw texts. And $w_d(b, e)$ denotes a subsequence which starts at the character position b and ends at the character position e.

The word embedding lookup table is defined as Eq. 4.12.

$$x_{b,e}^d = embed(w_d(b, e)) \tag{4.12}$$

where *embed* represents the same word embedding lookup table, and *b*, *e* represent the length between the prefix and the end of the word. Then the position spans are encoded by using sine and cosine functions of different frequencies as follows.

$$P_d^{2k} = \sin(d_{b,e}/10{,}000^{2k/d \bmod el}) \tag{4.13}$$

$$P_d^{2k+1} = \cos(d_{b,e}/10{,}000^{2k/d \bmod el}) \tag{4.14}$$

$$R_{b,e} = \mathrm{ReLU}(W_r P_d) \tag{4.15}$$

The final relative position code of the span is a learnable parameter, which replaces Eq. 4.10 with Eq. 4.16.

$$A_{b,e} = E_{x_i}^T W_q^T W_{k,E} E_{x_j} + E_{x_i}^T W_q^T W_{k,R} R_{b,e}$$
$$+ u^T W_{k,E} E_{x_j} + v^T W_{k,R} R_{b,e} \tag{4.16}$$

where W_q, $W_{k,E}$, $W_{k,R}$ are all learnable parameters.

According to the above relative position embedding, the hidden state can be calculated as Eq. 4.17.

$$h_i^l = Trm(h_i^{l-1}, A_{i,b,e}^{l-1}) \tag{4.17}$$

where h_i^l represents the embedding of the *i*th token, and the Transformer *Trm* which contains the multi-head attention layer, and/or the fully connected layer and/or the normalization layer, is the same as a normal Transformer in computing.

4.5 Multi-layer Soft Position Matching

For word segmentation information processing, there may be a variety of word segmentation situations of sentence segmentation in the Chinese environment. For example, "开放膀胱切开取石术" (open cystotomy and lithotomy) can be divided into the following scenarios such as "开放膀胱切开取石术" (open cystotomy and lithotomy), "开放/膀胱/切开/取石/术" (open/bladder/incision/lithotomy/surgery), "开放膀胱/切开/取石术" (open bladder/incision/lithotomy'), etc.

Because the word segmentation information is often a lexical boundary, it contains a large amount of the entity boundary information, and the choice of the word segmentation can affect the size of the entity information. Therefore, selecting the word segmentation is an important step of FLAT. The current format transformer is often a single-word segmentation situation, that is, it only introduces a single-word segmentation situation while ignoring other multiple-word segmentation situations. As a result, the format transformer cannot improve the recognition performance of medical named entities, which is far from improving the performance of Weibo, MSRA, and People's Daily datasets.

Therefore, the method of multi-layer soft location matching is firstly proposed in this work. That is, a dictionary, which contains commonly used medical terms and words, is established to achieve segmentation matching and select the optimized segmentation. When using the dictionaries to determine and select word segmentation, the dictionary matching conflicts will reduce the utilization of dictionary information.

Therefore, in order to solve the vocabulary matching conflicts, the soft matching algorithm is adapted in this work, whose advantages lie in the following facts.

(1) The problem of information loss can be avoided to a certain extent;
(2) It is convenient to change the model by introducing some word embedded information.

As shown in Fig. 4.6, Chinese sentence segmentation results may have multiple layers. Each layer of segmentation results is a sub-word with the different granularity, which may contain more sub-words with the different granularity. The importance of different sub-word results to the model locating entity span is different. The final performance of the obtained entity recognition depends on the fact that sub-word result is selected from the multi-level sub-word results. The purpose of multi-layer soft position matching is to select the splitting results. The word segmentation result, which is chose, determines the performance of the final entity recognition. For the above problem, the category and frequency of the word in the sub-word dictionary are used to get the scores of each sub word result, as shown in Eq. 4.18.

The sub-word matching result with the highest score is selected through the following softmax model (Fig. 4.7).

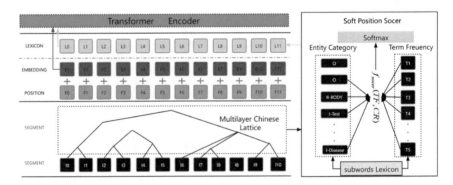

Fig. 4.6 Multilayer soft position matching module

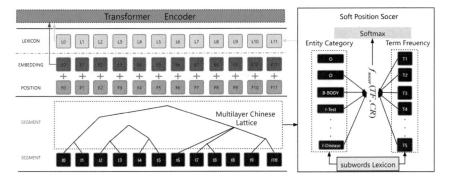

Fig. 4.7 Multilayer soft position word segmentation

$$f^i_{socer}(TF, CR) = TF \times CR = \sum_{i=0}^{L} \left(\frac{|x^i|}{N^i_c} * \frac{|x^i|}{x} \right) \tag{4.18}$$

where $TF = \frac{|x^i|}{N^i_c}$, $CR = \frac{|x^i|}{x}$, TF and CR represents the frequency of the segmentation and the category ratio of the word segmentation respectively, x^i is the number of occurrences of the sub-words, N^i_c is the total number of sub-words in the category, and x represents the number of occurrences in all categories.

Once the selected sub-word is determined, the sub-word is converted into the location information, which is used to fuse the vocabulary information. These ensures that the pretraining word embedding model can be used, and simultaneously minimizes the loss of information due to the word matching errors.

Some important advantages of this method lie in the following facts.

(1) This method eliminates the need to introduce vocabulary information in word embedding;
(2) This method gives full play to the parallel computing advantages of the model;
(3) This method improves the speed of model reasoning.

4.6 Fuzzy CRF

NER is essentially a labeling task for sequences. The labels of the sequence are not independent on each other, so it is necessary to deal with the relationship among the labels. Therefore, the CRF model, which is mainly adapted to decode NER in this section, has the following characteristics [4].

(1) the CRF model uses conditional probability as the basic principle to deal with the relationship among labels;
(2) the CRF model is suitable for labeling sequence data;
(3) the CRF can deal with mutually constrained relationship labels, and

(4)   the CRF model effectively solves the problem of sequence labeling.

When the neural network model is coded, the input of the CRF model is the output probability of the neural network model such as the BERT, the Transformer and etc., and the Viterbi algorithm is used to predict and find the global optimal annotation sequence.

After processing through the above procedures, an $n \times m$ matrix P is obtained, where n is the number of input words, m is the number of label types, $p_{i,j}$ is the probability that the label i of word j appears in the sentence, $x = \{x_1, \ldots, x_n\}$ denotes a sequence of sentences, $y = \{y_1, \ldots, y_i, \ldots, y_n\}$ does a sequence of labels, and $A_{i,j}$ is the transition probability from y_i to y_j. So, the corresponding score model is calculated as Eq. 4.19:

$$score(x, y) = \sum_{i-1}^{n} p_{i,y_i} + \sum_{i-1}^{n+1} A_{y_i-1y_i}$$

$$p(y|x) = \frac{\exp(score(x, y))}{\sum_y \exp(score(x, y))}$$

(4.19)

The corresponding objective function and the solution objective of CRF are Eqs. 4.20 and 4.21.

$$\min(\log P(y|x) = \min(score(x, y^x) - \log\left(\sum_{y'} \exp(score(x, y'))\right)$$ (4.20)

$$y^* = \arg\max(score(x, y'))$$ (4.21)

The total probability of all possible tag sequences, which is maximized by enumerating IOBES labels and all matching entity types [5], is defined as Eq. 4.22:

$$p(y|X) = \frac{\sum_{\bar{y} \in Y_p} \exp(score(x, \bar{y}))}{\sum_{\bar{y} \in Y_x} \exp(score(x, \bar{y}))}$$ (4.22)

where Y_x and Y_p denote all possible label sequences for the given sequence X and/or the modified IOBES scheme.

4.7 Experimental Setup and Simulation Results

4.7.1 Dataset

In order to prove the superiority of the proposed model in this chapter compared with traditional models, the proposed model and some related benchmark models are trained and evaluated on the 2019 CCKS dataset. In the 2019 CCKS-CNER dataset, there are six types of clinical entities that need to be identified, including diseases, image review, testing, treatment, drug, and anatomy. Several sentences in each piece of Chinese medical record data are annotated, which will result in a too long record if the whole sample record is not divided. Therefore, in order to limit the sentence length, each record is separated according to Chinese punctuation marks, and each Chinese sentence is treated in each record as a sample. Entities in Chinese texts are represented by "BIO", where "B", "I" and "O" respectively represent the beginning of the entity, the Chinese characters inside the entity and other irrelevant characters.

4.7.2 Pretrained Embedding and Modelling

Here, a lattice structure transformer called the entity recognition model is proposed, that can accurately capture the location of entities by combining sequences of characters with a pretrained model. The architecture of our model is shown in Fig. 4.8, which consists of four parts: the WordPiece module, the BERT module, the lattice structure Transformer module and the CRF module.

An overview of our methods is introduced as follows.

First, the WordPiece module is utilized to process the input text data to obtain the common medical terms and the common sequences of Chinese characters. Based on the above work, a medical clinic dictionary is established, which provides the lattice structure transformer layer with the position information of texts. Next, the BERT

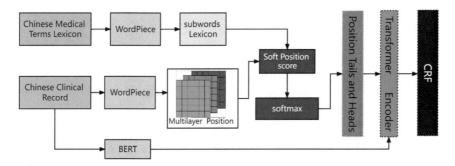

Fig. 4.8 The architecture of our proposed method

module is applied to convert the text into embedding and simultaneously captures the deep knowledge of the text, including part-of-speech, implicit language rules and major sentence features. Then, the CRF layer is used to legally decode the output of the previous modules and learns the constraints of labels. Finally, the output of CRF is the sequence labels.

The specific functions and underlying principles of each module are described in the following sub-sections.

(1) The BERT model is adapted to pretrain unlabeled Chinese clinical records provided by Li et al. [6] on the basis of 300-dimensional pretrained Chinese character embedding pretrained on Wiki texts.
(2) The BERT model has a total of 12 layer, each layer is the decoding part of the Transformer, and the number of the Transformer parameters at each layer is a self-attention layer with 512 input and output dimensions, and 8 attention heads. Since the maximum sequence length of the BERT is 512, the text sequences less than 512 lengths are performed to pad with zero and the text sequences longer than 512 lengths are truncated.
(3) The Adam optimization algorithm is used to train the language model during model training.
(4) The hardware is 2*GTX DELL T440 GPU.
(5) The initial learning rate is 6e−4, the epoch coefficient is 100, the batch is 10, the early stop is 25 to avoid overfitting.
(6) The learning rate is set to warm up in the first 50k steps, and the learning rate exhibits linear decay.
(7) A dropout probability 0.1 is used for all layers.
(8) This study uses python as the programming language.

The following section presents a visualization of the BERT's attention propagation in CNER. The colored squares in Fig. 4.9c represent one or more attention heads. The text in the Fig. 4.9 is the Chinese entities to be recognized in the clinical recorder. As can be seen from Fig. 4.9a, the line in the middle of Fig. 4.9a connects the Chinese characters on the left and right sides of Fig. 4.9a, representing the token's attention score. The saturation of the colors in Fig. 4.9c represents the intensity of attention.

4.7.3 Experimental Results

The results of the model proposed in this chapter and the baseline model on the CCKS 2019 dataset are shown in Table 4.3. The experimental results of the multi-layer soft position matching format Transformer entity automatic extraction model proposed in this chapter are in the last row of Table 4.3, namely the experimental results of BERT-Soft-Lattices-Transformer-fuzzy CRF. In the fourth and fifth rows of Table 4.3, BERT-LSTM-CRF and BERT-GRU-CRF respectively achieve better performance than the baseline without BERT, which further demonstrates the effectiveness of the BERT.

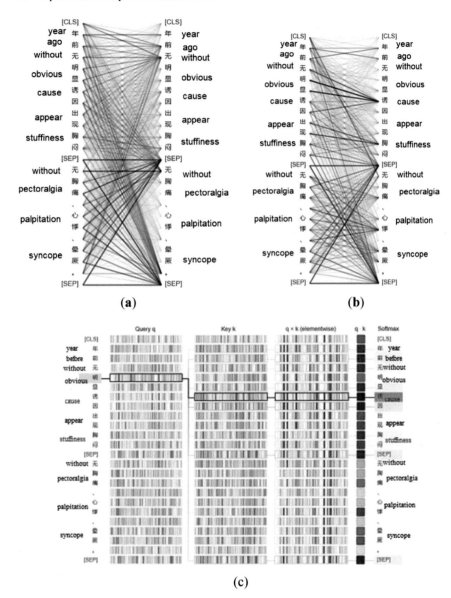

Fig. 4.9 BERT visualization: **a** attention-head view for BERT, for inputs. The left and center figures represent different layers/attention heads. The right figure depicts the same layer/head as the center figure, but with Sentence A → Sentence B filter selected; **b** model view of BERT, for same inputs, layers 4; **c** neuron view of BERT for layer 0, head 0

Table 4.3 Comparison of model performance

Models	P	R	F1	Cost time
BiLSTM-CRF	0.79	0.83	0.80	11 h
BiGRU-CRF	0.80	0.82	0.82	9 h 7 m
BERT-CRF	0.83	0.801	0.82	7 h 45 m
BERT-BiLSTM-CRF	0.86	0.91	0.88	8 h 32 m
BERT-BiGRU-CRF	0.85	0.86	0.85	7 h 23 m
BERT-FLAT-CRF	0.85	0.85	0.87	6 h 6 m
BERT-FLAT-fuzzyCRF [7]	0.868	0.83	0.793	6 h 10 m
BERT-Soft-Lattices-Transformer-fuzzyCRF	0.878	0.903	0.905	6 h 7 m

By augmenting the model with a word grid structure, the proposed model achieved a precision 0.878, a recall 0.90, an F1 score 0.905 and a model training time 367 min. The above results show that the proposed model achieves the performance of the BERT-LSTM-CRF model. While all losses are a small (almost negligible) improvement, and the cost-time performance is minimal too. Overall, the results illustrate the superior prediction performance of our method in CNER.

The general trends for epoch and F1 are provided in Fig. 4.8. Namely the relationship between epoch and F1 in the four models is presented. It can be easily concluded in Fig. 4.8 that the training time of the proposed model in this chapter and one of the BERT-FLAT-CRF are the least among all NER models, with training time 6 h 6 min, respectively. The proposed model reducing time consumption is due to the use of the Transformer and the word format structures, which facilitates parallel computing. Similarly, the reason of BERT-FLAT-CRF is because FLAT is also suitable for paralleling computing, and at the same time the computational complexity of CRF is much smaller than that of fuzzy CRF.

To sum up, the proposed multi-layer soft position matching format Transformer entity automatic extraction model (BERT-Soft-Lattices-Transformer-CRF) recognition has better recognition results and less time consumption.

4.7.4   Experiment Analysis

In recent years, the BiLSTM and the CRF have achieved excellent results in the NER tasks. However, in the clinical and medical application, providing interpretive information in Chinese medical records is critical to reduce computational time and maintain good performances. In this chapter, the proposed model, which is composed of the BERT module, the multi-layer soft position matching module, the word grid Transformer module and the fuzzy CRF module, can combine the powerful functions of the BERT and well-designed vocabulary word segmentation information. The proposed models make it possible for well-designed vocabulary word segmentation information, and strongly accelerated data trained parallelism.

Previous studies have shown that Chinese characters processing based on LSTMs are helpful in identifying clinical entities. Nonetheless, the models based on LSTM networks with CRF usually ignore some word information and the latent words. Some of the reasons have been given that these methods for CNER are not significantly different from English NER, and there exist some challenges for CNER. It is well known that encoding Chinese words in sentences can reduce the error propagation of word segmentation while exploiting word information.

Since Chinese words are applied as the case-form to encode the word information in the proposed model, which has a stronger ability to capture contextual information by using the word grid Transformer, and is easier to model long-distance dependencies. Therefore, it can also play the same role as the LSTM in exploring more distinct entity classes in various sentences. In addition, when recognizing thousands of Chinese characters, there always exists the risks that Chinese characters cannot be found in the sentence, and results in some negative recognition. Since the Transformer with a lattice-like Chinese character structure can capture the potential relevance among Chinese characters and phrases, this risk of recognition errors decreases.

From Fig. 4.10, it can be concluded that the constructed BERT model improves the accuracy of CNER, whose reason is to combine the BERT model with the BiLSTM-CRF, and can solve both negative and speculative detection problems.

In Table 4.3, the effect of the BERT model is better than that of the model without the BERT, which also proves that the BERT is beneficial to improve the accuracy of

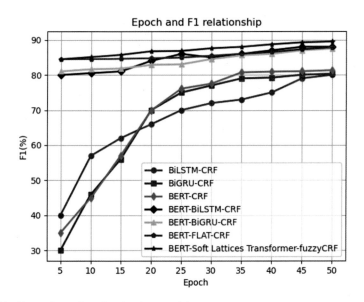

Fig. 4.10 Comparison of results of various models

the CNER. In addition, the fuzzy CRF can effectively deal with the existence of some entities in the NER annotation corresponding to multiple types of entity annotations, and reduces the error propagation caused by them.

Another advantage of the presented methods is their efficient accurate inference, whose role is forcefully to identify rare medical entities, because a direct and concise position encoding and a lattice Transformer plane are presented instead of using the LSTM. Simultaneously, the Transformer with parallel computing mechanism is used to reduce the model operation time, which is an effective way to reduce computation time and training time. Similarly, the residual networks and the self-attention mechanisms are typical parallelized models, which have been shown to have the advantage of fast computation in the NER [8, 9]. What needs to be pointed out is that both the proposed Transformer and the proposed word grid structure in this chapter have the similar characteristics. First, the proposed Transformer structure includes the residual network and the self-attention. Although the proposed Transformer is more complex, its multi-head self-attention, which has also a parallel computing mechanism, reduces the Transformer's run time. In addition, the proposed word grid structure is flattened, whose disadvantages of low computing performances and parallel inability are avoided.

4.8 Conclusion

In this chapter, an automatic entity extraction model of the Multi-layer Soft Position Matching Format Transformer is proposed. The word grid Transformer is used instead of LSTM to improve NER performances and the operation speed. Since LSTM has always been a key part of the NER model, the main reason is the ability of LSTM to capture contextual information, but because LSTM is a deep model of time series, there is a challenge of long computing time. In order to speed up the model operation, a different deep learning model is proposed, which replaces the LSTM neural network and also has the ability of capturing contextual information and less computing time. The experimental results of the proposed model also show that the multi-layer soft position matching format Transformer layer can achieve the similar performance of LSTM, while its precision, recall and F1 scores are 0.878, 0.903, and 0.905, respectively, which are higher than ones of other baseline models. These show that the multi-layer soft position matching format Transformer entity automatic extraction model has the same ability to capture contextual relevance as LSTM. It is worth noting that the proposed Transformer models is trained with the parallel computing mechanism, so the required training time is reduced, and a large amount of text data is processed in less time. The above experimental results also depict the advantage of this model in terms of the operation speed.

References

1. Sennrich R, Haddow B, Birch A. Neural machine translation of rare words with subword units. In: Proceedings of the 54th annual meeting of the Association for Computational Linguistics. 2016. p. 1715–25.
2. Lai Y, Liu Y, Feng Y, et al. Lattice-BERT: leveraging multi-granularity representations in Chinese pre-trained language models. In: Annual conference of the North American chapter of the Association for Computational Linguistics NAACL-HLT. 2021.
3. Li X, Yan H, Qiu X, Huang X. FLAT: Chinese NER using flat-lattice transformer. In: Proceedings of the 58th annual meeting of the Association for Computational Linguistics, online: ACL. 2020. p. 6836–42.
4. Lafferty J, McCallum A, Pereira FCN. Conditional random fields: probabilistic models for segmenting and labeling sequence data. In: The eighteenth international conference on machine learning ICML, Williamstown. 2001. p. 282–9.
5. Yan H, Deng B, Li X, Qiu X. TENER: adapting transformer encoder for named entity recognition. Comput Sci. 2019;342–441.
6. Li Y, Liu L, Shi S. Empirical analysis of unlabeled entity problem in named entity recognition. Int Conf Learn Representations. 2020;5(4):343–9.
7. Qin QL, Zhao S, Liu CM. A BERT-BiGRU-CRF model for entity re electronic medical records. Complexity. 2021;2021:1–11.
8. Zhang Z, Zhou T, Zhang Y, Pang YL. Attention-based deep residual learning network for entity relation extraction in Chinese EMRs. BMC Med Inform Decis Mak. 2019;19(2):171–7.
9. Yin M, Mou C, Xiong K, Ren J. Chinese clinical named entity recognition with radical-level feature and self-attention mechanism. J Biomed Inform. 2019;98:103289.

Chapter 5
Medical Named Entity Recognition Modelling Based on Remote Monitoring and Denoising

5.1 A General Framework

The electronic medical records (EMRs) are used in the public data set provided by Yidu Cloud to obtain remote data sets through remote supervision. For the obtained remote data set, in order to improve the reliability of the data set, the PU learning is adapted for denoising to reduce the negative impacts of mislabeled negative samples or unlabeled samples of the model. Finally, the negative samples and the pretraining models are used to extract a cancer information.

The whole research frame is shown in Fig. 5.1. This subsection simply describes some methods and strategies proposed in this chapter. Our approach focuses on reducing the dependence of the proposed model on data standards. The whole frame is divided into three parts as follows:

(1) The EMRs are used for remote supervision to obtain remote data sets;
(2) The positive and the unlabeled learning and the negative sampling are used to reduce the influence of standard errors on the obtained model;
(3) The BERT-MLP model is used to extract the entity information.

5.2 Research Targeted Problems

For the NLP, the lack of data is an important limitation for training models, especially in the fields of biology and medicine. The MNE involves many professional terms and terminologies, and requires professional practitioners to label, which is time-consuming, labor-intensive and costly. Therefore, the lack of data is the main challenge currently faced by the biomedical NER. And using remote supervision to solve the problem of insufficient data and data annotation has become the focus in the field of the NER. However, remote supervision often leads to data annotation errors, which has a large amount of noise effects on the final performance of the model. For example, only 20% of the samples belonging to a certain category are marked in

© The Author(s), under exclusive license to Springer Nature Singapore Pte Ltd. 2023   69
S. Guo et al., *Clinical Chinese Named Entity Recognition in Natural Language Processing*, https://doi.org/10.1007/978-981-99-2665-7_5

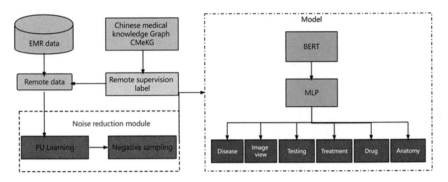

Fig. 5.1 Medical named entity recognition for remote monitoring/denoising

the data set, while the remaining 80% of the unlabeled samples contain the samples belonging to this category and the samples not belonging to this category. How to deal with incorrect labels of positive samples and negative samples is a challenge that needs to be solved, and the appropriate noise elimination algorithms need to be proposed to reduce the impact of error annotations on the above model.

5.3   Methods

5.3.1   Positive Sample and Unlabeled Learning Based on Category Risk Prediction

In a real life, it is not always possible or necessary to label good data samples. On many cases, it is difficult to obtain the negative samples, and it is because that the negative ones are too diversified and dynamic, only the positive samples and a large number of the unlabeled samples are available. A PU Learning is first used in the recommendation system, where there are often the positive samples clicked by users. Because the locations of the samples may be very biased, and the users do not click, it is impossible to identify whether the non-clicked users are negative samples or positive samples.

In this chapter, the PU learning algorithm is adapted to consider the category risk prediction. Here the PU learning is a research direction of semi-supervised learning, which refers to train a binary classifier in the case of only the positive and unlabeled data. At present, there are two solutions to the PU learning: one is that reliable negative samples are heuristically found from the unlabeled samples to train the binary classifier. The key ideas of this method are that the classification effect depends heavily on a prior knowledge; the other is that the unlabeled samples are used as the negative samples to train classification because the negative samples contain the positive samples, the wrong label assignment easily leads to classification errors. For the above model training, it is involved the Positive samples, the unlabeled learning bagging algorithm (PU Bagging) and the Two Step Approach.

The PU Bagging is a parallelization method. First, random subsamples from multiple unlabeled samples are extracted, which are used as the training data interactively to form multiple sets of a weak classifier. Each random training sample corresponds to a classifier, which outputs the score of each sample.

The Two Step Approach is different from the PU Bagging. First, a standard classifier of the positive samples and unlabeled samples will be trained. Second, the classifier is used to obtain a certain probability range of positive samples. Then, the negative samples with a greater certainty are marked according to the prediction probability, and the second classifier is trained on the relabeled data set. Finally, the process is repeated until the accuracy error is stable or a certain number of training times are reached. In this chapter, the PU learning is considered so that the dictionary does not need to label every data, and even requires to label all samples, which greatly reduces the requirements of the dictionary quality. Therefore, the use of the PU learning label corpus is relatively small in biology or medicine.

According to the latter method, a new loss function training model is proposed combined with the prediction risk function in this chapter, as shown in Fig. 5.2. The proposed model is continuously trained until minimizing the loss function according to the divided sub data sets, and simultaneously, the LSTM, a stable neural network are used as the PU classifiers.

First, each entity is classified into multiple binary classifications with positive samples and negative samples. The probability of positive classes is obtained by using neural networks such as the BiLSTM, and then the positive class is selected

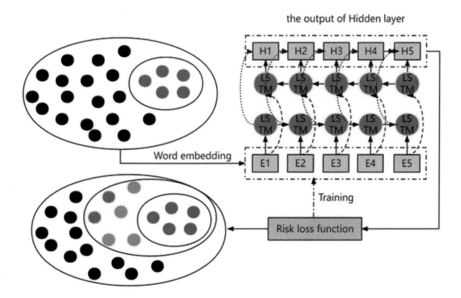

Fig. 5.2 Positive sample and unlabeled learning technology roadmap

with the highest probability as the word class. And further the BiLSTM is used to obtain the bidirectional hidden state, as shown in Eq. 5.1.

$$\vec{h}_t, \overleftarrow{h}_t = LSTM(e_t) \tag{5.1}$$

Secondly, through the probability of the positive class of the hidden layer state, the probability of the positive class is obtained by calculating the hidden state in Eqs. 5.2, 5.3 and 5.1.

$$e(w_t|s) = [\vec{h}_t \oplus \overleftarrow{h}_t] \tag{5.2}$$

$$f(w|s) = \delta\left(w_p^T e(w|s) + b\right) \tag{5.3}$$

Finally, the model is trained through the loss function defined by combing the predicted risk in Eq. 5.4 with the classification of each entity.

$$\hat{R}_\ell(f) = \gamma \pi_p \hat{R}_p^+(f) + \max\left\{0, \hat{R}_u^-(f) - \pi_p \hat{R}_p^-(f)\right\} \tag{5.4}$$

$$\hat{R}_p^+(f) = \frac{1}{|D^+|} \sum_{w|s \in D^+} \ell(f(w|s), 1) \tag{5.5}$$

$$\hat{R}_p^-(f) = 1 - \hat{R}_p^+(f) \tag{5.6}$$

$$\overset{-}{\hat{R}_u}(f) = \frac{1}{|D^u|} \sum_{w|s \in D^u} \ell(f(w|s), 0) \tag{5.7}$$

where π_p represents the proportion of unlabeled positive entities, D_e does a dictionary of entities for a given entity type, D_+ does as a set of labeled entity words, and the remaining unlabeled words does as D_u.

The predicted risk is defined as Eq. 5.8.

$$\ell(f(w|s), y) = |y - f(w|s)| \tag{5.8}$$

The creation of the binary classifier is completed by the above procedures. Since different classifiers are sent to each entity type, there exist multiple classification predictions for the same entity word. In general, the positive class with the highest probability is chosen as the class of the word. And the empirical risk of the labeled positive data is adapted to estimate the expected risk of positive data, and further some classical methods such as AdaSampling [1], etc. are utilized to expand the entity dictionary.

5.3.2 Negative Sampling Based on Positive/Negative Entity Probabilities

Negative samples are the process of selecting negative samples from the unlabeled data according to a certain strategy. They are mostly used for model training to speed up model training, which is an important feature to detect the model quickly.

The known unlabeled instances or the missing entities will definitely reduce the performance of the model. For this problem, a negative sampling method is proposed, namely, the partly unlabeled spans are randomly selected as the negative instances and the probabilities of positive and negative sample are adapted to calculate the training loss in this chapter. All negative instance candidates are obtained from the above data set. A subset is uniformly sampled from the entire candidate set. Finally, the span cross-entropy loss is obtained to train by Eq. 5.9.

$$\left(\sum_{(i,j,l)\in y} -\log\left(o_{i,j}[l]\right) \right) + \left(\sum_{(i',j',l')\in \hat{y}} -\left(p'_{pu} \log\left(o_{i',j'}[l']\right) + (1 - p_{pu})\log\left(o_{i,j}[l]\right) \right) \right)$$

$$(5.9)$$

where y is the negative entity sample set, $\hat{y}$ is the negative instance candidate set which belongs to the subset y, o is the probability of the non-entity label, p_{pu} is the prediction probability of the positive/negative instances of the sample by the PU learning in Sect. 5.3.1, and l is the model parameter.

The loss is trained by the negative sampling through adding some randomness, and thus the risk of the entity annotation quality is reduced. However, because the span loss function is simply the sum and subtraction of the probabilities of each subset, negative sampling is still unable to further reduce noise. In order to enhance the robustness of the training model, the above loss function is further improved and the symmetric attribute of the loss function is used to enhance the robustness of the model. Here the noises refer to samples with incorrect labels. The denoising is an unavoidable challenge in data labeling, especially for data obtained through remote supervision, where the noises occupy a larger proportion. The symmetric noise [2] means that all samples will be mislabeled as other labels with the same probability, and similarly, the asymmetric noises refer to different types of samples, and their probability of mislabel is also different.

According to the above concepts, the noise resistance of loss functions means that if a loss function is affected by noises, its risk minimization model is the same as the model trained by the noiseless data set.

Assume that the loss function of the model is $\sum_{i=1}^{k} L(f(x), i)$, and the category of the classification question is not empty. If the above loss function satisfies Eq. 5.10, it is said to be symmetric, as shown in Eq. 5.10.

$$\sum_{i=1}^{k} L(f(x), i) = C, \forall x \in \aleph, \forall f$$

$$(5.10)$$

where C is a constant.

Loss functions with symmetric properties are also more resistant to noise. Even when the noise is symmetric, the loss function is theoretically completely noise-resistant.

The proof process of this conclusion is as follows:

For a given model, assuming the symmetrical noise with the noise ratio η, the objective function R_L without noise, the objective function R_L^{η} with noise, and the expectations of the loss function on all training samples are shown as Eqs. 5.11 and 5.12.

$$R_L(f) = E_{X, y_x} L(f(x), y_x) \tag{5.11}$$

$$R_L^{\eta}(f) = E_{X, \hat{y}_x} L\big(f(x), \hat{y}_x\big) \tag{5.12}$$

If the loss function R_L^{η} is symmetric, it is easily the derivation of Eq. 5.13:

$$\begin{aligned}
R_L^{\eta}(f) &= E_{X, \hat{y}_x} L\big(f(X), \hat{y}_x\big) \\
&= E_X E_{y_x|X} E_{\hat{y}_x|X, y_x} L\big(f(x), \hat{y}_x\big) \\
&= E_X E_{y_x|X} \left[(1 - \eta) L(f(x), y_x) + \frac{\eta}{k - 1} \sum_{i \neq y_x} L(f(x), i) \right] \\
&= (1 - \eta) R_L(f) + \frac{\eta}{k - 1} (C - R_L(f)) \\
&= \frac{C\eta}{k - 1} + \left(1 - \frac{\eta k}{k - 1} \right) R_L(f) \\
&= A + \alpha R_L(f)
\end{aligned} \tag{5.13}$$

where $A = \frac{C\eta}{k-1}, \alpha = 1 - \frac{\eta k}{k-1}, i \neq y_x$ are the labels that are assigned to other classes by errors. It can be seen from the above that when $\alpha > 0$, R_L^{η} and R_L are linear dependence, if the optimal solution is the same, only the noise ratio of symmetric noise needs to be satisfied.

Therefore, the span loss function of negative sampling is introduced into the number of classifications. When it is large, the expected variable part of the loss function gradually decreases, and the loss function is closer to a constant. Therefore, the symmetric noises of the samples are utilized to enhance the robustness of the model.

5.3.3 Encoding Modelling

In this chapter, the BERT is used as an encoder to mitigate the effects on the image of annotated entities. The BERT is a transformer-based pretrained model, which is mainly applied to the specific NLP tasks through pretraining and fine tuning. In this experiment, the BERT [3], which is pretrained on a large-scale Chinese biomedical corpus, is used. The corpus covers Chinese medical Q&A, the Chinese medical encyclopedia and the Chinese electronic medical record.

Firstly, the pretrained BERT is used as an encoder to reduce the impact of annotated entities, and a hidden representation of each token is obtained, as shown in Eq. 5.14.

$$[h_1, h_2, \ldots, h_n] = BERT(e) \tag{5.14}$$

Then, the representation of each word is then obtained by the column-vector concatenation and the element-wise vector product, as shown in Eq. 5.15.

$$o_{i,j} = soft \max\left(W \tanh\left(U \tanh\left(W_h \cdot \left(h_i \oplus h_j \oplus \left(h_i - h_j\right) \oplus \left(h_i \cdot h_j\right)\right)\right)\right)\right) \tag{5.15}$$

Finally, a multilayer perceptron (MLP) is used to compute the label distribution.

5.4 Experimental Setup and Simulation Results

5.4.1 Datasets

The data set of this chapter is divided into remote data sets and gold data sets. The settings are the same as those described in Sect. 4.4.1, and the remote data sets are entity dictionaries extracted from the Chinese Medical Knowledge Graph (CMeKG). The entity dictionary extracted in this experiment contains 2554 entities, and the unlabeled data set is labeled with a matching algorithm to obtain a remote data set. The obtained data set contains a large number of incompletely annotated sentences, so it will naturally be troubled by the unlabeled entities. The gold data set is a well-marked data set through manual annotation and manual verification. Both data sets contain the same 20,000 human-annotated sentences.

In order to better verify the effectiveness of the model, 60% of remote data sets and the data samples of gold data sets are used as the remote supervision data training sets and the gold data training sets; The 50% data samples of the gold data set are randomly deleted and labeled to form artificial noise data training set; the remaining 40% of the gold data set is used as validation sets and test sets.

5.4.2 Experimental Setup

The same neural network super parameter configuration is used for all data sets. For example, L2 regularization and dropout ratio are respectively set to 1×10^{-5} and 0.4 to reduce the overfitting. The PU learning module mainly adopts the LSTM, with a dimension 256, a ratio λ 0.35. When the sentence encoder is the LSTM, whose hidden dimension is set to 512, and whose word representation is initialized by using pretrained word embedding. Here, Adam is used as the optimization algorithm and the recommended super parameters are adopted. During the evaluation, the prediction of the proposed model will be converted to the IOB format, and the conlleval script will be used to calculate the F1 score. In all above experiments, the proposed baseline models also use the above super parameter settings.

5.4.3 Simulation/Experiments Results

In order to illustrate the prediction effect of the PU learning on positive/negative samples, the experiments are conducted on the artificial noise data sets, and the unlabeled positive samples are identified using the PU learning. The experimental results show that PU learning can judge positive/negative entities of each entity category as shown in the following figures. The effects of the PU learning from Fig. 5.3a–f are respectively shown on positive/negative entities of each type of entity (disease, image inspection, test, treatment, medicine, anatomy). The recall rates of disease, image inspection, detection, surgery, medicine, and anatomical positions are respectively 73.3%, 82%, 90.3%, 27%, 74%, and 67%, five rates of which is 17–40% higher than ones of the methods using a dictionary (covering 50% of entities) and the time performance is the smallest. According to the proportion of various entities in the total samples, it can be demonstrated that PU learning can reduce the number of unlabeled samples to 23.5%.

The experiments are carried out on several entities to verify the effectiveness of the proposed method. The above experiments on artificial noise data sets show that the proposed model can identify unlabeled entities in training data, and simultaneously reduce unlabeled entities in data. The PU learning method adapted in the experiment has made significant improvement over dictionary matching. The experimental results also prove that the PU learning method used in the experiment can initially reduce the number of unlabeled negative samples in noisy and unlabeled data sets. In addition, the proposed model obtains the probability that each entity is a positive sample, which provides a basis for the next negative sampling.

Table 5.1 shows the results of model training on the artificial noise data training set and testing on the gold data test set. It can be verified that the proposed methods are obviously superior to the previous baseline model and achieves the most advanced performance.

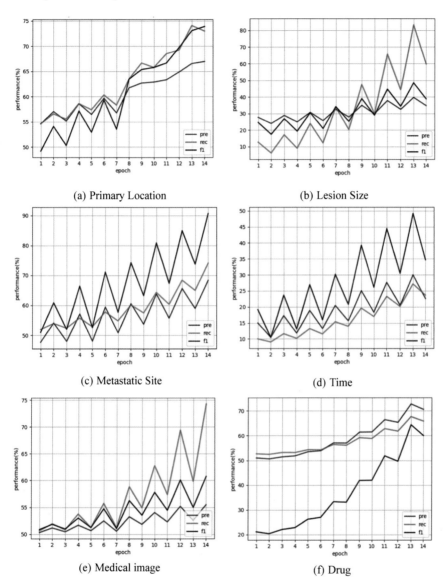

Fig. 5.3 Effect diagram of PU learning prediction positive sample

Table 5.2 shows the NER comparison results of the BERT-CRF trained on the gold data set and the PU-NA-BERT (PU-negative sampling BERT) trained on the artificial noise data set. The F1 of the PU-NA-BERT trained on the artificial noise data set is only 1.7% lower than one of the BERT-CRF trained on the gold data set. In addition, the gap between the two in precision and recall is 2.7 and 9.7%. Therefore, the above experimental results show that the PU-negative sampling method can make

Table 5.1 Comparison of noise data performance of 4 methods

Entity class	Model											
	BiLSTM-CRF			BERT-CRF			BERT-BiLSTM-CRF			PU-NA-BERT		
	Precision	Recall	F1	Precision	Recall	F1	Precision	Recall	F1	Precision	Recall	F1
Primary location	58.6	55.6	53.2	50.9	56.4	56.2	56.3	58.4	60.3	77.6	71.6	79.6
Size of lesion	55.2	50.2	54.7	56.3	57.8	53.4	54.1	59.5	61.4	75.6	75.4	74.7
Metastatic site	50.2	56.5	65.8	53.6	54.5	54.5	53.2	62.1	60.3	80.5	80.7	80.4
Time	56.54	54.5	51.3	56.8	58.6	51.2	57.5	60.4	65.6	77.3	83.5	77.3
Medical image	55.3	55.7	55.7	58.4	58.3	50.7	55.4	58.5	67.4	82.5	76.4	79.3
Drug	53.4	53.2	50.3	55.7	50.2	55.6	55.1	55.2	65.2	76.3	85.2	82.0
All entities	54.8	52.3	54.6	56.3	56.5	53.2	56.8	60.2	61.3	77.6	73.7	78.6

the training effect of noisy data sets close to the gold data sets. The purpose of this experiment is to show that the effect of noise data set training can be close to the gold data set through the PU negative sampling, so that the proposed model can no longer rely too much on high-quality labeled data sets, and high performance can also be achieved on the data sets that cover noises. Therefore, it can be seen that the proposed methods in this chapter can effectively reduce the errors caused by unmarked entities during model training.

Table 5.3 is the training on the remote data training set and testing on the gold data set. It can be seen from Table 5.3 that the proposed method still possesses great advantages. Compared with the baseline model, its effect has been greatly improved.

Table 5.4 is for training and testing on well annotated gold data sets. The proposed model still possesses the certain advantages, especially in the prediction of entity types with fewer samples, its performance is more outstanding.

In order to more directly show the negative effects of noise labels and negative samples, the performance of the proposed model on each data sets are shown through the loss function of the proposed model and F1 scores, as shown in Fig. 5.4.

For Fig. 5.4, it shows that in the model training stage, by using the PU learning and the negative sampling, the training model in the noise data set can be as close as possible to the model in the gold data set. The loss convergence of the trained model in the gold data set is faster, while the loss convergence of the trained model in the noise data set is slower. The red line denotes the loss of the trained model in the noise data set, whose declined amplitude is far less than the loss of the gold data set training. It further shows that the model needs to spend more time to learn when training the model on the noise data. In order to fit the large loss caused by noise points, the models often lead to learn error information guides, which also leads to the model learning noise sample ability worse than their learning the "correct label". However, in the model using the PU learning and the negative sampling, the decreasing trend of the loss is closer to the loss of gold trained data sets. The blue line in the Fig. 5.4 lies between the red line and the black line, which means that the proposed model can be unbiased and consistently estimate the task loss. In a conclusion, its effect is like completely-labeled data sets. For the model using the PU negative BERT sampling, the effects in the remote labeling data set and the artificial noise data set are better than those of other baseline models.

These simulation results show the following facts.

(1) The PU learning can effectively be used to reduce the impact of annotation quality on the proposed model;

Table 5.2 Comparison of the performance of BERT-CRF trained on the golden dataset and PU-negative sampling-BERT trained on artificial noise dataset

BERT-CRF trained on the gold dataset			PU-negative sampling-BERT trained on artificial noise dataset		
Precision	Recall	F1	Precision	Recall	F1
80.3	83.4	80.3	77.6	73.7	78.6

Table 5.3 Performances of the baseline and our models on the remote training data set

Entity class	Model											
	BiLSTM-CRF			BERT-CRF			BERT-BiLSTM-CRF			PU-negative sampling-BERT		
	Precision	Recall	F_1	Precision	Recall	F_1	Precision	Recall	F_1	Precision	Recall	F_1
Primary location	68.52	45.46	35.4	65.45	43.23	37.4	65.06	44.17	47.1	66.78	52.31	48.8
Size of lesion	57.53	30.45	42.3	60.38	27.45	38.3	58.43	31.27	45.3	64.43	48.75	50.3
Metastatic site	54.56	33.23	32.5	64.06	35.75	36.0	64.59	34.56	45.7	65.34	56.57	47.6
Time	63.12	39.43	45.4	63.12	45.37	46.5	65.71	57.16	55.1	67.20	60.22	58.1
Medical image	65.23	42.32	27.3	75.23	40.59	32.1	68.13	53.33	35.2	74.32	57.88	65.0
Drug	57.55	30.98	28.7	57.19	34.41	35.2	62.34	38.56	45.2	67.56	62.81	54.0
All entities	63.04	43.77	34.1	59.14	40.32	36.1	61.19	57.53	55.4	65.54	61.18	63.2

Table 5.4 Performance comparison of each model on the gold data

Entity class	BiLSTM-CRF		BERT-CRF		BERT-BiLSTM-CRF		PU-negative sampling-BERT	
	Recall	F1	Recall	F1	Recall	F1	Recall	F1
Disease	83.34	88.7	87.04	87.3	88.45	91.3	79.40	76.3
Image	66.2	68.4	62.5	70.3	65.4	70.3	82.4	77.4
Inspection	70.32	65.1	65.5	67.2	75.7	67.2	80.5	74.1
Treatment	81.03	78.5	80.33	82.3	83.4	79.5	71.60	5.76
Medicine	71.3	66.9	74.8	65.4	64.8	65.4	78.4	71.1
Primary location	82.4	87.2	63.8	71.1	86.9	87.4	5.85	2.23
The whole entity	90.84	90.3	95.84	91.3	93.21	88.5	92.39	88.7

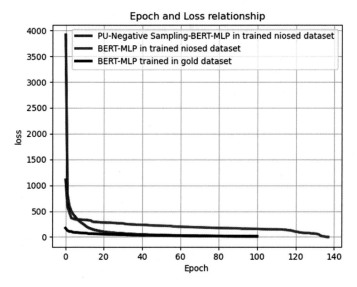

Fig. 5.4 Training loss model

(2) Negative sampling can further limit the performance degradation caused by unlabeled samples.

(3) The pretrained BERT model is more suitable for remote supervision as a cancer information extraction model.

By using the PU learning and lexicon matching, a remotely denoised supervision approach is adapted to obtain remote datasets, and similarly by using negative sampling and the pretrained model, the impact of incorrect annotation is reduced, thus the data that lacks annotation or has little manual annotation, can achieve good performances.

In this chapter, we also present the baseline methods based on the LSTM, the GRU, and the BERT, and do some experiments on the golden dataset, and finally find that the proposed method can meet or exceed the performance of other models both on the golden dataset and on the remote dataset. For example, the proposed method can effectively extract a primary tumor location, a tumor size, and a metastasis location on the cancer clinical records lacking annotation, with an F_1 score of 90%. In addition, many performances such as the impact of dictionary size, the PU learning balance rate are evaluated.

The main reason that the model misidentifies the entities is due to the lack of labeled data and the treatment of unlabeled data as negative samples. Aiming at the impact of few entity samples caused by the lack of labeled data, the use of pretrained models is adopted to alleviate this pressure. In the Tables 5.3 and 5.4, the methods with the pretrained BERT model are higher than those without the BERT. Aiming at the problem that unlabeled data seriously misleads the model during model training and greatly affects the performance of the model, this chapter uses the PU learning to identify unlabeled entities in the training data, and depends on the probability that negative sampling is defined as the positive sample, and further reduce the negative impact on the model.

Compared with other models, the performance on the gold dataset is not outstanding, but the performance on a small number of medical entities is higher than one on the baseline model, which also shows that this method has a more prominent ability to mine the entities with few samples.

5.5 Conclusions

This chapter uses the EMR data in the public data set provided by Yidu Cloud to obtain remote data sets through remote supervision. In order to improve the reliability of the data set, the PU learning is used to denoise the obtained remote data set to reduce the negative impact of mislabeled negative samples or unlabeled samples on the proposed model. Finally, the entity information extraction and classification are performed using negative sampling and a pretrained model. The experimental results show that the used remote-supervised denoising method and pretrained model can achieve more than 60% F_1 score on both the remote data set and the noise data set. Compared with the medical NER model, the proposed method in this chapter has the best recognition performance while requiring the lowest annotation quality of the dataset. In conclusion, for EMR data sets that contain noise, denoising remote supervision methods can improve the performance of models for extracting entity information from EMRs, while alleviating the model's dependence on high-quality datasets. Therefore, the proposed methods have the potential to reduce labor costs and improve clinical decision-making systems.

References

1. Yang P, Ormerod JT, Liu W, Ma C, Zomaya AY. AdaSampling for positive-unlabeled and label noise learning with bioinformatics applications. IEEE Trans Cybern. 2018;49(5):1932–43.
2. Shang J, Liu L, Gu X, et al. Learning named entity tagger using domain-specific dictionary. In: 2018 Conference on empirical methods in natural language processing EMNLP, Brussels. 2018. p. 342–53.
3. Zhang X, Zhang Y, Zhang Q, Ren Y, Qiu TL, Ma JH. Extracting comprehensive clinical information for breast cancer using deep learning methods. Int J Med Informatics. 2019;132: 103985.

Outlook

In this work, the Chinese MNE is taken as the research direction, and the historical research development and the current status for the medical NER are summarized. Based on the current research status and challenges faced by the Medical Named Entity Recognition (MNER) such as enhancing the model context capture ability, improving the location information perception ability of the pretrained model, and identifying/denoising the unlabeled entities. The following proposed methods such as the LSTM neural network medical NER model with the parameter sharing unit, the multi-layer soft position matching format Transformer entity automatic extraction model, and the PU learning methods under negative sampling denoising are proposed, correspondingly.

The main research contents and innovations of this work are as follows:

(1) For the improvement of the LSTM neural network model, by adding parameter sharing units towards the LSTM, the long-distance dependency problem of the LSTM is improved and the ability to capture context information are enhanced too. The parameter sharing units can not only learn shared parameters from a given task, but also realize learning and training across a certain sequence length. Therefore, it is proposed that the LSTM variant neural networks with shared parameters not only span a wider range of contexts, but also contain a richer text information. The simulation results show that the effects of long text medical entity recognition have been greatly improved.

(2) In order to achieve the following purposes: strengthening BERT's ability to perceive location information, studying the influence of self-attention mechanism on location information, improving Transformer by using Chinese subword grid results, enhancing the model's ability to learn location information, and reducing its ability to weaken location information. Based on these factors, a multi-layer soft location matching format Transformer entity automatic extraction model is proposed, and the following functions are achieved through the method proposed in this work: the soft location matching score selects the best word segmentation scheme, the word and word sequence information is

S. Guo et al., *Clinical Chinese Named Entity Recognition in Natural Language Processing*, https://doi.org/10.1007/978-981-99-2665-7

directly introduced through the multi granularity word grid to introduce the position representation of the Transformer, and the Transformer uses the fully connected self-attention mechanism to learn the long-distance dependencies of the sequence.

(3) For the noise problem caused by the characteristics of medical data sets in the NER task, the PU learning, the negative sampling and the pretrained model are used to reduce the impact of noise on the model. The combination of the PU learning and the negative sampling is proposed to train unlabeled entities to eliminate errors caused by the unlabeled entities, and reduces the dependence of the model on text annotation in this work.

The purpose of Chinese MNER is to automatically identify effective entities from clinical medical records or medical texts, and then classify the entities to achieve sequence annotation. Chinese MNER is an important part of smart medicine, which is conducive to mine the information hidden in medical texts, so as to provide medical entity information for clinical medical decision-making and medical research. Although the MNER has made great progress, it still faces challenges such as poor robustness, poor generalization, dependence on data quality, and data imbalance. Due to the limitation of computational force and insufficient time, the research work still needs to be improved. Future researches and experiments will focus on the following aspects:

(1) The improvement of the NER recognition effect of the LSTM variant neural network model with parameter sharing unit should be further verified by mathematical proof or more experiments. In addition, the parameter sharing unit shall be combined with other neural networks (GRU, RNN etc.) to verify the improvement effect of its recognition results

(2) Multilayer soft position matching format Transformer entity automatic extraction model uses subword grid results that need word segmentation, and the word segmentation method is based on dictionary matching. This part of the research should carry out more experiments on the influence of dictionaries, so as to determine the influence of dictionaries on the final recognition effect.

(3) For the use of the PU learning method in MNER for noise removal and remote supervision, it is necessary to set the different parameters, and the super parameters have a great impact on the final experimental results. The slight difference in the super parameters setting will lead to huge differences in the experimental results. In addition, it is useless to get the relationship between the super parameters and the experimental results through multiple experiments. Future research meetings should summarize the impact of super parameters or design the PU learning methods to reduce the impact of super parameters.

Appendix

Tables A.1, A.2, A.3.

Table A.1 Performance comparison table of each model on noise data

Category of medical entity	BiLSTM-CRF			BERT-CRF			BERT-BiLSTM-CRF			PU-negative-BERT		
	Accuracy	Recall	F1	Accuracy	Recall	F1	Accuracy	Recall	F1	Accuracy	Recall	F1
Disease	58.6	55.6	50.9	50.9	56.4	56.2	56.3	58.4	60.3	77.6	71.6	79.6
Image	55.2	50.2	54.7	56.3	57.8	53.4	54.1	59.5	61.4	75.6	75.4	74.7
Test	50.2	56.5	65.8	53.6	54.5	54.5	53.2	62.1	60.3	80.5	80.7	80.4
Treatment	56.54	54.5	51.3	56.8	58.6	51.2	57.5	60.4	65.6	77.3	83.5	77.3
Medicine	55.3	55.7	55.7	58.4	58.3	50.7	55.4	58.5	67.4	82.5	76.4	79.3
Site	53.4	53.2	50.3	55.7	50.2	55.6	55.1	55.2	65.2	76.3	85.2	82.0
Whole entity	54.8	52.3	54.6	56.3	56.5	56.8	56.8	60.2	61.3	77.6	73.7	78.6

Table A.2 Performance comparison table of each model on remote data

Category of medical entity	BiLSTM-CRF			BERT-CRF			BERT-BiLSTM-CRF			PU-negative-BERT		
	Accuracy	Recall	F1	Accuracy	Recall	F1	Accuracy	Recall	F1	Accuracy	Recall	F1
Disease	68.52	45.46	35.4	65.45	43.23	37.4	65.06	44.17	47.1	66.78	52.31	48.8
Image	57.53	30.45	42.3	60.38	27.45	38.3	58.43	31.27	45.3	64.43	48.75	50.3
Test	54.56	33.23	32.5	64.06	35.75	36.0	64.59	34.56	45.7	65.34	56.57	47.6
Treatment	63.12	39.43	45.4	63.12	45.37	46.5	65.71	57.16	55.1	67.20	60.22	58.1
Medicine	65.23	43.32	27.3	75.23	40.59	32.1	68.13	53.33	35.2	74.32	57.88	65.0
Site	57.55	30.98	28.7	57.19	34.41	35.2	62.34	38.56	45.2	67.56	62.81	54.0
Whole entity	63.04	43.77	59.14	59.14	40.32	36.1	61.19	57.53	55.4	65.54	61.18	63.2

Table A.3 Performance comparison table of each model on gold data

Category of medical entity	BiLSTM-CRF			BERT-CRF			BERT-BiLSTM-CRF			PU-negative-BERT		
	Accuracy	Recall	F1	Accuracy	Recall	F1	Accuracy	Recall	F1	Accuracy	Recall	F1
Disease	87.54	83.34	88.7	90.21	87.04	87.3	95.24	88.45	91.3	85.56	79.40	76.3
Image	72.12	66.2	68.4	70.31	62.5	70.3	74.31	65.4	70.3	76.4	82.4	77.4
Test	77.04	70.32	65.1	76.62	65.5	67.2	77.52	75.7	67.2	75.6	80.5	74.1
Treatment	85.4	81.03	78.5	88.43	80.33	82.3	89.44	83.4	79.5	81.16	71.6	5.76
Medicine	75.43	71.3	66.9	73.12	74.8	65.4	73.22	64.8	65.4	81.3	78.4	71.1
Site	76.7	82.4	87.2	83.6	63.8	71.1	90.04	86.9	87.4	73.30	5.85	2.23
Whole entity	95.4	90.84	90.3	89.20	95.84	91.3	88.45	93.21	88.5	87.31	92.39	88.7

Printed in the United States
by Baker & Taylor Publisher Services